30 YEARS YOUNGER

THE 6 EVIDENCE-BASED HABITS OF BIOLOGICAL AGE REVERSAL

DR. K.D. CHRISTENSEN

CONTENTS

Introduction 5

1. Habit 1: Nutrition & Diet for Biological Age Reversal 9
2. Habit 2: Exercise and Movement for a Youthful Body 29
3. Habit 3: Cultivating Healthy Relationships and Activities 43
4. Habit 4: Mastering Sleep for Cellular Regeneration 59
5. Habit 5: Managing Stress for Longevity 73
6. Habit 6: 10 Primary Biological Age Factors That Are Understood To Be Reversible 87
7. Bonus Habit: Integrating Age-Reversing Habits into Daily Life 105

Conclusion 119

References 123

INTRODUCTION

What if I told you that your true age isn't the number of candles on your birthday cake? That the wear and tear on your body, the very essence of how young or old you feel, can be measured, and more importantly, reversed? This is the groundbreaking science of biological age reversal, and it's not just a far-fetched dream—it's a reality that you can start embracing today.

In this book, we'll dive deep into the cutting-edge research that proves one revolutionary truth: aging is not an irreversible process. Your biological age, a measure of how your body is actually functioning, can be turned back, giving you the vitality, energy, and health of someone decades younger. The key lies in adopting six specific, evidence-based habits that have been shown to rewind the clock on a cellular level.

But what exactly is biological age, and how does it differ from the chronological age we're all familiar with? While chronological age is simply the number of years you've been alive, biological age is a more accurate reflection of your body's true condition. It considers factors like the health of your cells, the length of your telomeres (the protective caps on your DNA), and the accumulation of damaging processes like inflammation and oxidative stress. In essence, it's a snapshot of how well your body is functioning, and it can be measured through advanced tests like the Index Test from Elysium Health, considered the gold standard in determining biological age.

Throughout this book, we'll explore the six core habits that have been scientifically proven to reverse biological age: nutrition and diet, exercise, cultivating healthy activities and relationships, sleep, managing stress, and incorporating specific age-reversing nutrients. Each of these habits is backed by rigorous research and studies, and when combined, they create a powerful blueprint for turning back the clock on aging.

But this isn't just an abstract concept—it's a reality that I, Dr. K.D. Christensen, have experienced firsthand. As a retired healthcare wellness provider with over 40 years of experience, I've dedicated my life to understanding and implementing these evidence-based habits. And the results speak for themselves. On March 7th, 2023, at the chronological age of 70, my biological age measured by the Index Test was just 58 years old. But the transformation didn't stop there. By fully embracing Habit 6 for an entire year, I was able to further reduce my biological age. At 72 years old, my Index Test revealed a biological age of only 42—a stunning 30-year reversal.

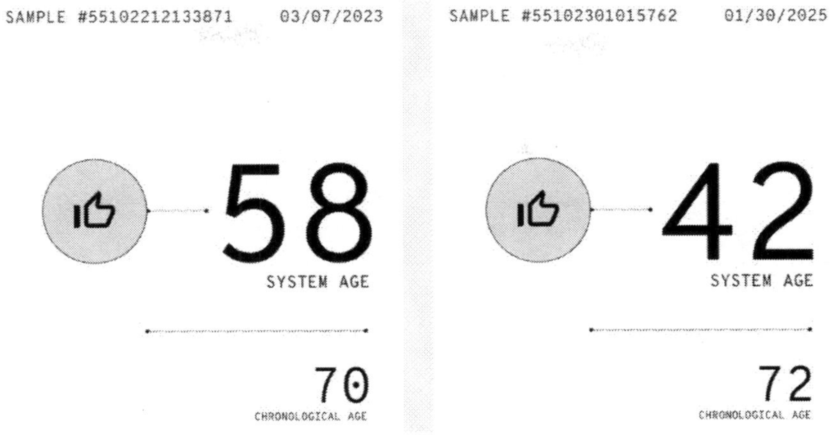

Fig. Index Test from Elysium Health

This book is structured to guide you through each of these transformative habits, providing not only the scientific underpinnings but also practical strategies for incorporating them into your daily life. Whether you're in your 30s, 50s, or beyond, it's never too early or too late to start your journey towards a younger, healthier you.

By the end of this book, you'll be equipped with the knowledge and tools to take control of your biological age, to feel younger, more energetic, and more vibrant than you ever thought possible. You'll understand how to nourish your body with the right foods, how to optimize your exercise routine for maximum age-reversal benefits, how to cultivate the relationships and activities that keep you young, and so much more.

But more than that, you'll be empowered to rewrite your aging story. You'll see that getting older doesn't have to mean a decline in health and vitality—that with the right habits, you can turn back the clock and experience a level of wellbeing you never knew was possible.

So let's embark on this transformative journey together. Let's explore the science, the strategies, and the secrets to unlocking a younger, healthier you. The path to reversing your biological age starts here, and I couldn't be more excited to guide you every step of the way.

1

HABIT 1: NUTRITION & DIET FOR BIOLOGICAL AGE REVERSAL

Have you ever wondered why two people of the same age can look and feel so different? The secret often lies not in their genes, but in what they eat. This chapter reveals how your diet is a powerful tool in your quest to reverse biological aging. From the complex interactions of nutrients with your DNA to the personalized choices that optimize health, we'll explore how what you consume can transform how you age. Nutrition is not just about feeding your body; it's about feeding your genes and, ultimately, your youth.

UNDERSTANDING NUTRIGENOMICS: HOW FOOD INTERACTS WITH GENES

Nutrigenomics, a burgeoning field at the intersection of nutrition and genetics, delves into how the foods you eat can influence gene expression. It's not just about the calories or macronutrients; it's about how these elements interact with your DNA to either accelerate or decelerate the aging process. Epigenetic modifications, such as DNA methylation, provide a framework for understanding how dietary choices can influence gene activity without altering the genetic code itself. Nutrients like folate and B vitamins are key players here, as they contribute to the methylation process, potentially impacting everything from inflammation to cancer risk, as indicated by studies in the field (Source 1). By understanding and harnessing these interactions, you can tailor your diet to promote longevity and vitality.

The interplay between specific nutrients and gene expression is profound. Omega-3 fatty acids, found in abundance in foods like flaxseeds and salmon, have been shown to modulate inflammatory gene expression, reducing the chronic inflammation that often accompanies aging. Polyphenols, abundant in berries and green tea, activate antioxidant pathways that protect your cells from oxidative stress, a major contributor to aging. These nutrients essentially act as switches, turning beneficial genes on and harmful genes off. This gene-diet interaction is a key aspect of nutrigenomics, highlighting the potential of diet to influence your biological age.

Personalized nutrition, which involves tailoring dietary choices based on individual genetic profiles, represents the future of nutritional science. With nutrigenetic testing, you can gain insights into how your body responds to certain foods and nutrients, allowing for more targeted dietary recommendations. For instance, some individuals may benefit from a diet rich in leafy greens and cruciferous vegetables, which are known to support detoxification pathways and provide a plethora of bioactive compounds beneficial for cellular health. Others might find fermented foods, rich in probiotics, to be particularly effective in maintaining gut health and supporting immune function.

To help you apply these concepts, consider incorporating gene-friendly foods into your diet. Increasing your intake of leafy greens and cruciferous vegetables, such as kale and broccoli, can provide your body with essential nutrients needed for optimal gene expression. Fermented foods like kimchi and yogurt can enhance your gut microbiome, which in turn can influence your overall health and longevity. By making these changes, you support your biological age reversal and lay the groundwork for a healthier future.

THE POWER OF PLANT-BASED ANTIOXIDANTS IN AGE REVERSAL

Antioxidants serve as the body's defense against oxidative stress, a process that accelerates aging by producing harmful molecules known as reactive oxygen species (ROS). These unstable molecules damage cells, proteins, and DNA, which can hasten the onset of age-related conditions. By neutralizing ROS, antioxidants help maintain cellular integrity and promote longevity. The role of antioxidants is thus pivotal in not only slowing aging, but also in supporting overall health. As you age, understanding the impact of these compounds becomes increasingly crucial, offering a natural means to mitigate the effects of time on your body.

Among the most potent plant-based antioxidants are flavonoids, catechins, and resveratrol, each found in everyday foods. Flavonoids, abundant in berries like blueberries and strawberries, offer a rich source of compounds that combat oxidative stress. Catechins, primarily found in green tea, provide powerful protective effects against cellular damage. Resveratrol, present in red grapes is celebrated for its potential in reducing inflammation and extending lifespan. Incorporating these antioxidants into your diet can help fortify your body's defenses. Not only do they fight the ravages of aging, but they also contribute to overall wellbeing by supporting heart health and cognitive function.

Antioxidants play a critical role in cellular repair and protection. They aid in detoxifying cells by removing harmful substances, thereby enhancing the body's natural repair mechanisms. This includes repairing DNA damage, which, if left unchecked, can lead to premature aging and disease. By maintaining the health of your cells, antioxidants support tissue regeneration and help preserve youthful function. Integrating antioxidant-rich foods into your meals can provide your body with the tools it needs to repair itself. This dietary approach can significantly influence how effectively your body combats the signs of aging.

ANTIOXIDANT-RICH RECIPES TO TRY

To easily include these powerful compounds in your diet, consider starting your day with a berry smoothie packed with spinach. Blend together a handful of blueberries, strawberries, and a cup of spinach with a splash of almond milk for a refreshing, nutrient-dense breakfast. For lunch, a herb tea and citrus salad can be both satisfying and healthful. Brew a cup of herb tea, let it cool, and use it as a base for a dressing with lemon juice and olive oil. Toss it with mixed greens, orange slices, and walnuts. These meals taste great and deliver a hearty dose of antioxidants to support your body's fight against aging.

INTERMITTENT FASTING: TIMING YOUR MEALS FOR MAXIMUM IMPACT

Intermittent fasting is more than just a dietary trend; it's a scientifically backed approach that can significantly impact metabolic health and longevity. By strategically timing your meals, intermittent fasting influences various physiological processes that contribute to age reversal. The concept revolves around periods of eating and fasting, allowing your body to enter a state of autophagy. This is a natural process where the body cleanses itself of damaged cells and regenerates new ones, crucial for maintaining youthful cellular function. Additionally, intermittent fasting has been shown to improve insulin sensitivity, which plays a vital role in reducing the risk of age-related diseases like diabetes and cardiovascular disorders. This method of eating optimizes how your body uses energy and supports a healthier, more vibrant life.

There are several approaches to intermittent fasting, each offering unique benefits and flexibility. The 16/8 method is perhaps the most popular, where you fast for 16 hours and eat during an 8-hour window, typically from noon to 8 p.m. This method aligns easily with social and work life, making it a sustainable choice for many. Another approach, known as Eat-Stop-Eat, involves fasting for a full 24 hours once a month or as often as twice a week. While more intense, it allows for greater flexibility on non-fasting days. Both methods encourage the body to shift from glucose metabolism to using fat and ketones for energy, a shift that can enhance performance and slow aging. These fasting regimens help in weight management and support long-term health benefits.

The benefits of intermittent fasting extend beyond weight control. Fasting increases human growth hormone levels, which aid in muscle growth, fat loss, and overall cellular repair. Furthermore, it reduces chronic inflammation, a key player in the aging process. By lowering inflammation, fasting helps mitigate its damaging effects on tissues and organs. For those new to fasting, gradual initiation is recommended. Start by extending your overnight fast by an hour or two, gradually working up to your desired fasting window. During fasting periods, staying hydrated is crucial. Water, herbal teas, and black coffee can help maintain hydration without breaking the fast. Timing your nutrient intake is also important; focus on nutrient-dense meals during eating windows to ensure you're meeting your body's needs without overeating.

HARNESSING THE BENEFITS OF FERMENTED FOODS FOR GUT HEALTH

The gut, often referred to as the body's second brain, plays a pivotal role in overall health, influencing everything from immunity to mood. A healthy gut microbiome is essential for biological age reversal, as it maintains balance and supports efficient bodily functions. Diversity within your gut microbiota is crucial because a varied microbiome can fend off pathogens, synthesize essential nutrients, and regulate inflammation. Fermented foods, teeming with beneficial bacteria, are a natural way to enhance this diversity. These foods help cultivate a robust microbial community, which can significantly impact how your body ages.

Fermented foods like kimchi and sauerkraut are not only delicious but also rich in probiotics, which are live bacteria that confer health benefits. These foods support gut health by replenishing and balancing the gut flora, which can be disrupted by poor diet, stress, or antibiotics. Probiotics in fermented foods help improve digestion, boost the immune system, and may even contribute to weight management. Kefir, another potent fermented food, is packed with prebiotic fibers that feed the good bacteria in your gut, promoting their growth and activity. Regular consumption of these foods can create an environment in your gut that supports age reversal by keeping harmful bacteria at bay and promoting overall health.

Among the myriad of fermented foods, some stand out for their specific benefits. Kombucha, a fermented tea, is renowned for its detoxifying properties, aiding the liver in processing toxins and improving energy levels. Miso soup, a staple in Japanese cuisine, is not only comforting but also filled with immune-boosting compounds, supporting your body's natural defenses. Incorporating these foods into your diet doesn't require drastic changes. A simple yogurt parfait, layered with nuts and seeds, can serve as a nutritious breakfast or snack, delivering a hearty dose of probiotics. For meals, a tempeh stir-fry with vegetables offers a protein-rich, flavorful dish that supports gut health. By adding these foods to your daily routine, you can enhance your gut microbiome and contribute to a more youthful biological age.

SUPERFOODS AND THEIR ROLE IN CELLULAR REPAIR

The term "superfoods" has become ubiquitous in discussions about health and wellness, yet its significance goes far beyond buzzwords. These are foods distinguished by their exceptionally high nutrient density and antioxidant capacity. They offer concentrated sources of vitamins, minerals, and phytochemicals that can support cellular health and repair. This is crucial as our cells face daily assaults from free radicals and environmental stressors. Superfoods provide the body with the necessary tools to combat these challenges, fostering resilience and vitality at the cellular level. They serve as a cornerstone for dietary strategies aimed at reversing biological age.

Among the myriad of superfoods, a few stand out for their profound impact on cellular repair and longevity. Spirulina, a blue-green algae, is renowned for its detoxifying properties, helping the body eliminate toxins while providing a rich source of protein and essential amino acids. Chia seeds, tiny yet mighty, are packed with omega-3 fatty acids, which play a vital role in maintaining cell membrane integrity and reducing inflammation. Acai berries, celebrated for their anti-inflammatory properties, are rich in antioxidants that protect cells from oxidative damage. These superfoods bolster cellular health and contribute to a diet that supports long-term wellbeing and youthfulness.

The science behind superfoods lies in their unique ability to activate sirtuins, a class of proteins that regulate cellular health and longevity. Sirtuins play a crucial role in enhancing mitochondrial function, which is vital for energy production and overall cellular efficiency. By supporting mitochondrial health, superfoods help maintain the body's energy levels and delay the onset of age-related decline. This intricate interaction highlights the importance of integrating these foods into your diet. They don't just nourish the body; they optimize cellular operations, paving the way for improved health and extended lifespan.

Incorporating superfoods into your daily meals can be straightforward and enjoyable. Start your day with a smoothie bowl enriched with spirulina, blending it with your favorite fruits and a splash of almond milk for a nutritious breakfast. For a mid-day treat, consider a chia seed pudding mixed with almond milk and topped with fresh fruits. These simple yet effective recipes enhance your diet and provide your cells with the necessary nutrients to repair and thrive.

BLUE ZONE SECRETS: LONGEVITY DIETS FROM AROUND THE WORLD

Blue Zones are regions where people live significantly longer and healthier lives, not by chance, but through a combination of lifestyle habits that have been passed down through generations. These areas, including Okinawa in Japan, Sardinia in Italy, and Ikaria in Greece, boast high concentrations of centenarians, individuals who live to be 100 years or older. The common thread among these regions is a lifestyle that includes a strong sense of community, low stress levels, regular physical activity, and, crucially, a diet rich in plant-based foods. These elements create a blueprint for longevity that can be emulated by anyone willing to make similar lifestyle changes.

The dietary habits observed in Blue Zones offer a fascinating glimpse into how food choices impact longevity. In Okinawa, diets are predominantly plant-based, featuring a variety of vegetables, tofu, and sweet potatoes, which are a staple food known for their high nutrient content and antioxidant properties. Sardinia, meanwhile, embraces the principles of the Mediterranean diet, which emphasizes whole grains, legumes, and healthy fats from sources like olive oil. This diet is also rich in omega-3 fatty acids from fish and nuts, providing heart health benefits and supporting cognitive function. Each of these dietary patterns is low in processed foods and red meat, reducing the intake of harmful fats and additives.

Unique foods from these regions play a crucial role in promoting longevity. In Okinawa, for example, sweet potatoes are not only a dietary staple but also a rich source of vitamins and fiber, contributing to the overall health and vitality of the population. Similarly, the residents of Ikaria regularly consume wild greens, which are packed with phytochemicals and antioxidants. These foods support immune function and help reduce the risk of chronic diseases. By incorporating such nutrient-dense foods, individuals can mimic the benefits experienced by those living in Blue Zones, potentially extending their own healthspan.

Adapting Blue Zone principles into your own life can be straightforward. Start by increasing the amount of vegetables and legumes in your meals, aiming for a variety of colors and types to maximize nutrient intake. Incorporate healthy fats from sources like avocados and nuts, and consider replacing red meat with fish or plant proteins. Emphasize whole, unprocessed foods, and aim to make meals a social event, enjoying them with family or friends to enhance emotional wellbeing. By adopting these simple, yet powerful dietary habits, you can take a significant step towards a longer, healthier life.

THE ROLE OF OMEGA-3 FATTY ACIDS IN CELLULAR HEALTH

Omega-3 fatty acids are crucial for maintaining cellular health, and they come in three primary forms: Eicosapentaenoic acid (EPA), Docosahexaenoic acid (DHA), and Alpha-linolenic acid (ALA). EPA and DHA, found predominantly in marine sources like salmon and mackerel, play a vital role in reducing inflammation and supporting brain function. ALA, on the other hand, is found in plant sources such as flaxseeds and chia seeds. Our bodies convert ALA into EPA and DHA, though not very efficiently, which is why direct consumption of these fatty acids is beneficial. Understanding their structure and sources can empower you to make informed dietary choices that support cellular integrity.

Omega-3s are integral to the structure of cell membranes, enhancing their fluidity and functionality. This fluidity is essential as it facilitates nutrient transport and waste elimination, thereby maintaining cellular efficiency. Moreover, omega-3s improve cellular communication by supporting the function of cell receptors, which play a role in cellular signaling processes. This improved communication is crucial for the proper functioning of the nervous system, cardiovascular health, and immune response. By incorporating omega-3 rich foods into your diet, you are effectively supporting the very foundation of your cellular health.

The benefits of omega-3s extend well beyond cellular maintenance. They have a profound impact on cardiovascular health by reducing triglycerides, lowering blood pressure, and decreasing the risk of heart disease. These fatty acids also support cognitive function, potentially slowing age-related cognitive decline and reducing the risk of neurodegenerative diseases. Research has shown that adequate intake of omega-3s can improve mood disorders, providing mental health benefits alongside physical ones. The comprehensive benefits underscore the importance of ensuring these fatty acids are a staple in your diet.

To reap the benefits of omega-3s, consider incorporating fatty fish like salmon and mackerel into your meals a few times a week. For those preferring plant-based options, flaxseeds and chia seeds are excellent sources of ALA. Alternatively, omega-3 supplements can offer a convenient way to meet your dietary needs, especially if your intake from natural sources is insufficient. Whether through diet or supplements, maintaining a steady intake of omega-3s can significantly contribute to your overall health and aid in reversing biological aging.

POLYPHENOLS: POTENT PLANT COMPOUNDS FOR LONGEVITY

Polyphenols are a diverse group of naturally occurring compounds found abundantly in plants, and they are classified into flavonoids, phenolic acids, and lignans. These compounds play a crucial role in the plant's defense mechanisms, and when consumed by humans, they offer a multitude of health benefits. Flavonoids, for example, are found in fruits, vegetables, and beverages like herbal tea, and they are known for their antioxidant properties. Phenolic acids are present in whole grains, while lignans are abundant in seeds and whole grains. Each class of polyphenols contributes uniquely to health, providing a broad spectrum of protective effects against diseases and aging.

The antioxidant and anti-inflammatory properties of polyphenols are central to their ability to combat oxidative stress and inflammation, two key factors in the aging process. These compounds work by scavenging free radicals, thereby neutralizing these harmful molecules before they can damage cells. Additionally, polyphenols inhibit the production of pro-inflammatory cytokines, thus reducing inflammation throughout the body. This dual action protects cellular structures and supports the body's natural healing processes, which can slow down the aging process and reduce the risk of chronic diseases.

Polyphenols also influence longevity-related signaling pathways, such as the activation of sirtuins and the modulation of AMPK and mTOR pathways. Sirtuins are proteins that regulate cellular health and have been linked to increased lifespan and improved metabolic efficiency. By activating these proteins, polyphenols enhance the body's ability to manage energy and repair damaged cells. Moreover, they modulate AMPK and mTOR pathways, which are involved in cellular growth and stress responses. This modulation helps maintain cellular homeostasis and promotes resilience against age-related decline, offering a promising strategy for extending health span.

Incorporating foods rich in polyphenols into your diet is a practical way to harness their benefits. Dark chocolate is a delicious source of flavonoids, offering a sweet way to support heart health and cognitive function. By including these foods in your daily meals, you can enhance your diet with powerful compounds that promote health and longevity.

THE ANTI-AGING EFFECTS OF VITAMIN D

Vitamin D, often dubbed the "sunshine vitamin," plays a pivotal role in maintaining health, particularly as we age. It is unique among vitamins because our bodies synthesize it when our skin is exposed to sunlight. This synthesis begins when ultraviolet rays from the sun trigger vitamin D production in the skin. Once synthesized, vitamin D undergoes two hydroxylations in the body for activation—first in the liver and then in the kidneys. Its primary role involves the regulation of calcium and phosphorus levels, crucial minerals for maintaining bone integrity and strength. Without adequate vitamin D, bones can become thin, brittle, or misshapen, leading to conditions such as osteoporosis. This vitamin's reach extends beyond bones, influencing various bodily systems, including the immune system.

The immune system benefits profoundly from vitamin D, which enhances innate immunity and modulates the immune response. This vitamin can reduce the risk of autoimmune diseases by dampening excessive immune responses that attack the body's tissues. Its role in supporting immune health is particularly important for older adults, whose immune systems naturally weaken with age. Ensuring sufficient vitamin D levels can help bolster defense mechanisms against infections and chronic illnesses, making it a vital component of an aging well strategy. Studies have shown that individuals with adequate vitamin D levels have a lower incidence of autoimmune disorders such as rheumatoid arthritis and multiple sclerosis, highlighting its protective role.

Vitamin D's impact on bone health is well-documented, yet its benefits for aging extend to muscle function as well. It aids in the maintenance of muscle strength, which is crucial for preventing falls and fractures in older adults. By supporting bone density and muscle integrity, vitamin D helps maintain mobility and independence as we age. To achieve optimal levels, consider regular sun exposure, aiming for about 10–30 minutes a few times a week, depending on skin type and location. Dietary sources such as fortified foods and fatty fish also contribute to vitamin D intake. If sunlight and diet are insufficient, supplements can ensure you meet the recommended levels, typically around 600-800 IU daily for adults, though individual needs may vary.

COENZYME Q10: ENERGIZING CELLS FOR YOUTHFULNESS

Coenzyme Q10, often abbreviated as CoQ10, is a naturally occurring antioxidant found in every cell of your body. It plays a crucial role in producing energy at the cellular level, primarily through its participation in the electron transport chain within the mitochondria. This process is vital for the synthesis of adenosine triphosphate (ATP), the energy currency of the cell. Without CoQ10, cells would struggle to maintain energy production, leading to fatigue and diminished cell function. Moreover, CoQ10 provides antioxidant protection by preventing lipid peroxidation, a damaging process where free radicals attack cell membranes, leading to cellular damage and aging.

The health of your mitochondria, often described as the powerhouses of the cell, is directly linked to CoQ10 levels. By supporting mitochondrial function, CoQ10 enhances ATP production, ensuring that cells have the energy they need to perform optimally. This helps in maintaining youthful vigor and reduces mitochondrial oxidative stress, which can lead to cellular dysfunction over time. Oxidative stress in mitochondria is a significant contributor to aging and various age-related diseases. By minimizing this stress, CoQ10 plays a protective role, promoting longevity and vitality.

CoQ10's benefits extend to cardiovascular health, where it plays a pivotal role in improving endothelial function. The endothelium, a thin membrane lining the inside of the heart and blood vessels, relies on CoQ10 to enhance its ability to relax and contract. This improved function can lead to lower blood pressure and better circulation, reducing the risk of cardiovascular diseases. Furthermore, CoQ10 helps in maintaining the elasticity of blood vessels, which can naturally stiffen with age, thereby supporting overall cardiovascular health.

Incorporating CoQ10 into your diet can be achieved through various sources. Organ meats such as liver and heart are rich in CoQ10, as are fatty fish like mackerel and sardines. For those who may not consume these foods regularly, CoQ10 supplements offer an alternative to ensure adequate intake. These supplements can be particularly beneficial for older adults, as natural CoQ10 production tends to decrease with age, making supplementation an effective strategy to maintain youthful cellular energy and function.

CURCUMIN AND ITS IMPACT ON INFLAMMATION AND AGING

Curcumin, the vibrant yellow compound found in turmeric, has garnered attention for its profound health benefits, particularly its anti-inflammatory properties. As the active ingredient in turmeric, curcumin is celebrated for its ability to combat inflammation at the molecular level, making it a potent ally in the fight against aging. The process of aging is closely linked to chronic inflammation, which acts like a slow-burning fire, damaging tissues and contributing to the development of age-related diseases. Curcumin works by inhibiting the activity of nuclear factor kappa-light-chain-enhancer of activated B cells (NF-kB), a protein complex that plays a critical role in regulating the immune response to infection. By suppressing NF-kB signaling, curcumin effectively reduces inflammation and protects the body's cells from the damage that accelerates aging. This ability to modulate inflammatory pathways showcases curcumin's potential as a natural anti-aging elixir.

Beyond NF-kB inhibition, curcumin also influences cytokine production, which are small proteins important in cell signaling. These proteins can either exacerbate or reduce inflammation, and curcumin exerts its benefits by tipping the balance in favor of anti-inflammatory cytokines. This modulation of cytokine activity offers significant implications for managing age-related diseases. For instance, in neurodegenerative conditions like Alzheimer's, where inflammation is a key component, curcumin's ability to reduce inflammation could lower the risk or slow the progression of these disorders. Similarly, its anti-inflammatory effects support joint health, offering relief to those suffering from arthritis, a common ailment associated with aging. By addressing the root causes of inflammation, curcumin alleviates symptoms and supports long-term health.

Despite its impressive properties, curcumin's bioavailability presents a challenge, as it is not easily absorbed into the bloodstream. To enhance absorption, pair curcumin with black pepper, which contains piperine, a compound shown to increase bioavailability by up to 2000%. Additionally, consuming curcumin with fats, such as those found in avocado or coconut oil, can further improve its uptake. These strategies ensure that the body can fully benefit from curcumin's anti-inflammatory and age-defying properties. Whether sprinkled on roasted vegetables or stirred into a warm curry, incorporating curcumin into your diet, alongside these absorption-enhancing methods, can be a practical step toward healthier aging.

ADAPTOGENS: NATURAL ALLIES IN STRESS REDUCTION

Adaptogens, a remarkable class of herbs and plants, have captivated the wellness community for their unique ability to bolster the body's resilience to stress. Unlike typical stimulants, adaptogens work by modulating the body's stress response, enhancing its ability to cope with anxiety and fatigue without causing overstimulation or burnout. These natural substances have been used for centuries in traditional medicine systems, such as Ayurveda and Traditional Chinese Medicine, and are now gaining recognition in modern wellness circles. Their properties enable the body to maintain balance and homeostasis, even in the face of stressors that threaten to disrupt hormonal equilibrium.

One of the key physiological benefits of adaptogens is their role in regulating cortisol levels. Cortisol, often dubbed the "stress hormone," is released in response to stress and plays a vital role in a host of bodily functions, including metabolism and immune response. However, chronic stress can lead to persistently elevated cortisol levels, which may contribute to a host of health issues, from weight gain to weakened immunity. Adaptogens help to normalize cortisol production, thus avoiding the damaging effects of prolonged stress. Moreover, they support adrenal health, ensuring that the adrenal glands, which produce cortisol, function optimally. This support is crucial for maintaining energy levels and overall vitality.

Among the most popular adaptogens are Ashwagandha, Rhodiola, and Holy Basil, each offering distinct benefits. Ashwagandha, revered in Ayurvedic medicine, is renowned for its ability to reduce stress and anxiety, while also promoting restful sleep. Rhodiola, a hardy plant that thrives in cold climates, is celebrated for enhancing mental clarity and combating fatigue, making it a favorite among those seeking cognitive support. Holy Basil, a staple in traditional Indian healing practices, is valued for its immune-boosting properties and ability to promote emotional balance. Together, these adaptogens offer a multifaceted approach to stress management, helping to fortify the body against the pressures of modern life.

Incorporating adaptogens into your routine can be simple and rewarding. Herbal teas and tinctures offer a soothing way to enjoy the benefits of these herbs, with blends tailored to specific needs, such as relaxation or mental focus. Adaptogenic supplements provide a convenient option for those looking to enhance their diet with these powerful plants. Whether consumed as a calming tea in the evening or as a supplement with breakfast, adaptogens can seamlessly integrate into your lifestyle, offering a natural means to enhance resilience and maintain balance. As you explore these natural allies, you'll discover a world of possibilities for nurturing your wellbeing and supporting your body's ability to thrive amidst stress.

WHAT TO AVOID

From a medical standpoint, avoiding tobacco, alcohol, caffeinated coffee, and tea is essential for optimal health and disease prevention. Tobacco use is a leading cause of cancer, cardiovascular disease, and respiratory conditions, with no safe level of exposure. Alcohol, even in moderate amounts, increases the risk of liver disease, hypertension, certain cancers, and cognitive decline. Caffeinated beverages like coffee and tea can contribute to sleep disturbances, increased heart rate, and dependency, particularly in individuals with cardiovascular conditions or anxiety disorders.

Eliminating these substances supports overall well-being, enhances immune function, and reduces the risk of chronic illnesses, promoting a healthier and more sustainable lifestyle.

2

HABIT 2: EXERCISE AND MOVEMENT FOR A YOUTHFUL BODY

Have you ever considered that the secret to staying young might lie not in the fountain of youth, but in the way you move your body each day? Exercise doesn't just tone your muscles or trim your waistline; it plays a fundamental role in keeping your body biologically young. This chapter will explore how exercise, particularly High-Intensity Interval Training (HIIT), can be a powerful tool in reversing the signs of aging and enhancing your overall vitality. Through strategic, focused movements, you can improve not only your physical health but also your cellular and metabolic functions, setting the stage for a more robust and energetic life.

High-Intensity Interval Training, or HIIT, is a form of exercise that alternates between short bursts of intense activity and periods of rest or low-intensity movement. The core principle of HIIT is to push your body to its maximum capacity during the high-intensity intervals, then allow it to recover during the rest periods. This design not only makes workouts shorter but also incredibly effective. The beauty of HIIT lies in its efficiency; you can achieve significant fitness gains in a fraction of the time compared to traditional exercise routines. HIIT workouts typically last anywhere from 15 to 30 minutes, making them ideal for those with busy schedules who still wish to reap the benefits of vigorous exercise.

The benefits of HIIT for aging are profound. Engaging in HIIT can lead to improvements in cardiovascular health, evidenced by enhanced insulin sensitivity and increased VO2 max, which is a measure of your body's ability to use oxygen during exercise. Enhanced insulin sensitivity helps your body use glucose more efficiently, reducing the risk of developing insulin resistance and type 2 diabetes. Similarly, an increased VO2 max reflects a higher level of aerobic fitness, which is associated with lower mortality rates and a longer lifespan. HIIT has also been shown to enhance mitochondrial function within skeletal muscle, a crucial factor in maintaining muscle energy and function as we age. This improvement in cellular energy production helps mitigate one of the major adverse effects of aging: the decline in muscle efficiency and strength.

Incorporating HIIT into your routine can be straightforward and adaptable to various fitness levels. A simple 20-minute circuit could include exercises like jumping jacks and burpees, alternating between 30 seconds of intense activity and 30 seconds of rest. For those seeking a structured approach, the Tabata protocol offers an effective format: 20 seconds of all-out effort followed by 10 seconds of rest, repeated for four minutes per exercise. This method can be applied to sprints and push-ups, offering a challenging yet rewarding workout. These routines maximize calorie burn and keep your metabolism elevated long after the workout ends, a phenomenon known as the afterburn effect.

Safety is paramount when engaging in HIIT, especially for beginners or individuals with limitations. It's essential to start with a gradual increase in intensity, allowing your body to adapt to the demands of high-intensity exercise. Listening to your body and avoiding pushing beyond your limits can prevent injuries. For those with joint concerns or who prefer a gentler approach, low-impact alternatives like cycling or rowing can provide the same benefits without the strain on joints. These modifications ensure that everyone, regardless of fitness level, can participate in and benefit from HIIT.

Interactive Element: Design Your HIIT Workout

Crafting a personalized HIIT routine can be both a fun and rewarding endeavor. Follow these steps to create a workout that suits your fitness level and goals:

1. **Select Your Exercises**: Choose 4-5 exercises that target different muscle groups. Examples include jumping jacks, squats, push-ups, and mountain climbers.
2. **Determine Your Interval Times**: Decide on the duration of your high-intensity and rest intervals. Beginners might start with 20 seconds of activity and 40 seconds of rest, while more advanced exercisers can try 30 seconds of activity and 30 seconds of rest.
3. **Plan Your Workout Duration**: Aim for a total workout time of 15 to 30 minutes, adjusting the number of sets and exercises based on your time availability.
4. **Gradually Increase Intensity**: As you become more comfortable with the routine, gradually increase the intensity by reducing rest times or increasing activity duration.

By designing a HIIT workout tailored to your needs, you can ensure that exercise becomes a sustainable and enjoyable part of your age-reversal strategy.

THE SCIENCE OF STRENGTH TRAINING FOR MUSCLE PRESERVATION

As we age, the importance of maintaining muscle mass becomes increasingly evident. Strength training emerges as a key player in preserving muscle health, a crucial aspect of metabolic wellness and longevity. One of the most significant benefits of strength training is its role in preventing sarcopenia—the age-related loss of muscle mass and strength. This condition can lead to frailty, reduced mobility, and increased risk of falls, making it imperative to address through targeted exercise. Regular strength training not only combats sarcopenia, but also boosts your basal metabolic rate, the number of calories your body burns at rest. This boost in metabolism helps manage weight and can counteract the gradual decline in metabolic efficiency that often accompanies aging. By engaging in strength training, you create a foundation for a healthier, more resilient body that can better withstand the challenges of aging.

Strength exercises can take many forms, each offering unique benefits tailored to different fitness goals and preferences. Resistance bands, for example, are excellent tools for enhancing flexibility and building strength without the need for heavy equipment. They provide variable resistance, which can be adjusted to suit individual fitness levels, and are especially beneficial for those new to strength training or looking for low-impact options. Weightlifting, on the other hand, is known for its profound impact on bone density. By placing controlled stress on bones, weightlifting stimulates bone growth and helps maintain bone strength, a critical factor in preventing osteoporosis. Incorporating a mix of resistance bands and weightlifting into your routine can create a balanced approach to strength training, one that supports both muscular and skeletal health.

Developing a personalized strength training plan is vital for achieving and maintaining muscle health. A well-structured plan often includes split routines, where different muscle groups are targeted on different days. This approach allows for adequate rest and recovery, preventing overtraining while ensuring each muscle group receives attention. Progressive overload, the gradual increase in resistance or intensity, is another essential technique. This method ensures continuous improvement by challenging muscles to adapt and grow stronger. Whether you're lifting free weights, using machines, or relying on body weight, consistency and progression are key. By crafting a plan that aligns with your lifestyle and goals, you can make strength training an integral part of your health regimen.

The mind-muscle connection is a concept that underscores the importance of focus and intention during workouts. This connection involves consciously engaging the muscles you're working on, enhancing the effectiveness of each exercise. Visualization techniques can be particularly beneficial, allowing you to mentally picture the muscle contracting and relaxing. This focus improves muscle activation and fosters a deeper understanding of your body's movements. Concentrating on form and posture is equally critical, as proper technique minimizes the risk of injury and maximizes the benefits of each exercise. By honing your attention on the task at hand, you cultivate a more mindful approach to strength training, one that supports both physical and mental well-being.

FLEXIBILITY AND BALANCE EXERCISES FOR LONGEVITY

Flexibility and balance are often overlooked, yet they are crucial components of a comprehensive fitness regimen, particularly as we age. These elements contribute to physical well-being and play a pivotal role in maintaining independence and preventing injuries. As we grow older, the risk of falls increases, posing significant threats to our health and autonomy. Engaging in exercises that enhance flexibility and balance helps mitigate this risk by improving coordination and stability. A well-stretched body allows for a greater range of motion, facilitating daily tasks and reducing the likelihood of strains or sprains. Furthermore, flexible muscles are less prone to injury, allowing you to move with ease and confidence. The ability to maintain your balance can mean the difference between a minor misstep and a serious fall, making these exercises indispensable in promoting longevity and quality of life.

To bolster your flexibility and balance, incorporating key exercises into your routine can yield profound benefits. Dynamic stretching routines, which involve moving parts of your body while gradually increasing reach and speed, are effective in enhancing flexibility and preparing your muscles for more strenuous activity. These stretches mimic the movements you perform in everyday life, making them particularly functional. Balance drills, such as single-leg stands, are equally crucial. By practicing standing on one leg, you challenge your body's equilibrium and strengthen the core muscles that stabilize you. This simple exercise can be adapted to various difficulty levels, making it accessible to individuals of all fitness backgrounds. Additionally, incorporating movements like walking heel-to-toe or practicing yoga poses, such as the tree pose, can further improve your balance and coordination.

Incorporating flexibility and balance exercises into your daily routine doesn't require a significant time commitment, yet it can have a lasting impact on your health. Starting your day with a morning stretch sequence can invigorate your muscles and mind, setting a positive tone for the day. Simple stretches like reaching for the sky, bending to touch your toes, or performing gentle twists can awaken your body and improve circulation. Balance practice can be seamlessly integrated into mundane activities, such as brushing your teeth. By standing on one leg while you brush, you can effortlessly work on your balance without adding extra time to your daily schedule. These small adjustments can cumulatively lead to substantial improvements in your flexibility and balance.

Beyond the physical advantages, flexibility and balance exercises offer significant mental health benefits. Engaging in mindful movement, where focus is placed on the sensations and mechanics of each motion, can effectively reduce stress and promote relaxation. This mindful approach encourages present-moment awareness, helping to quiet the mind and alleviate anxiety. The rhythmic nature of stretching and balance exercises can have a meditative effect, promoting a sense of calm and well-being. As stress levels decrease, you may find that your mood improves, leading to a more positive outlook on life. Moreover, the confidence gained from improved physical capabilities can translate to greater self-assuredness in daily activities. This holistic approach to fitness not only enhances your physical health but also nurtures your mental and emotional well-being, creating a balanced foundation for a healthier lifestyle.

LOW-IMPACT WORKOUTS FOR JOINT HEALTH

As we gracefully age, preserving the health of our joints becomes increasingly paramount. Low-impact exercises are those that put minimal stress on the joints while allowing you to engage in effective physical activity. This makes them an ideal choice for maintaining joint health and enhancing overall wellbeing. Unlike high-impact workouts that can strain ligaments and cartilage, low-impact exercises provide a gentler approach. They allow you to build endurance, improve cardiovascular health, and maintain muscle tone without the risk of joint damage. This is particularly beneficial for those with arthritis or other joint concerns, as these exercises can help reduce pain and stiffness, enabling you to stay active and enjoy a full range of motion throughout life.

Among the most effective low-impact activities, swimming stands out as a comprehensive workout that engages the entire body. The buoyancy of water supports your weight, significantly reducing the stress on joints while providing resistance that strengthens muscles. Swimming builds endurance and flexibility and improves heart health, making it an excellent choice for those looking to sustain their fitness levels without putting undue pressure on their joints. Cycling is another joint-friendly exercise that offers substantial cardiovascular benefits. Whether on a stationary bike or cycling outdoors, this activity allows you to enhance leg strength and improve stamina while keeping the impact on your knees and hips minimal. Both swimming and cycling can be adjusted in intensity to accommodate different fitness levels, ensuring that everyone can participate and reap the rewards.

Creating a low-impact workout plan requires thoughtful consideration of your current fitness level, goals, and schedule. A balanced routine might include swimming sessions a few times a week, where you alternate between different strokes to target various muscle groups. Incorporating resistance exercises with bands can further enhance muscle strength without the need for heavy weights. These bands provide adjustable resistance, allowing for a customized workout that challenges muscles while protecting joints. For those new to exercise or those with specific limitations, starting with shorter sessions and gradually increasing duration and intensity can help build confidence and stamina. Consistency is key, and maintaining a varied routine ensures that you address all aspects of fitness while keeping your workouts engaging.

The importance of proper footwear and equipment cannot be overstated when it comes to supporting joint health during physical activity. Investing in quality footwear with adequate cushioning can make a significant difference in comfort and performance, particularly for activities that involve standing or walking. Shoes designed with shock absorption help minimize the impact on your joints, reducing the risk of injuries. For those who engage in activities like cycling, ensuring that your bike is properly adjusted to your height and body mechanics can prevent strain and enhance efficiency. Additionally, using knee supports or braces can provide extra stability and protection, especially for individuals with existing joint issues. These simple yet effective measures can enhance your exercise experience, allowing you to move with confidence and ease.

Low-impact workouts offer a sustainable way to maintain fitness and overall health, especially as we age. They provide a gentle yet effective means of staying active, promoting not only joint health but also cardiovascular fitness, muscle strength, and mental well-being. By incorporating various activities and ensuring the use of appropriate equipment, you can enjoy the benefits of exercise without the worry of joint strain or injury. This approach supports your physical health and contributes to a balanced lifestyle that values movement, adaptability, and longevity. As you engage in these activities, you'll find that they enhance your physical capabilities and invigorate your spirit, providing a sense of accomplishment and wellbeing that permeates every aspect of life.

THE ROLE OF DAILY MOVEMENT: BEYOND THE GYM

Have you ever thought about how much movement you incorporate into your day outside the confines of structured exercise sessions? Many people focus intensely on hitting the gym, yet overlook the powerful impact of everyday activities on their overall health. This is where non-exercise activity thermogenesis, or NEAT, comes into play. NEAT encompasses all the little movements you perform throughout the day that aren't part of deliberate exercise routines—things like walking to the store, cleaning the house, or even fidgeting. These seemingly minor activities can significantly boost your daily calorie expenditure, supporting weight management and overall metabolic health. Increasing your NEAT can be as effective as a traditional workout in terms of energy expenditure. It's about making movement a natural part of your life, not just something you do at the gym.

Increasing daily movement doesn't require drastic changes. Simple strategies can integrate more activity into your routine, enhancing your NEAT. Consider taking the stairs instead of the elevator; it's a small choice that can have a big impact over time. Each step you take contributes to your heart health and leg strength without necessitating extra time in your schedule. Another effective tactic is transforming meetings into walking sessions. Walking meetings not only encourage physical activity but also stimulate creativity and collaboration. When you're on the move, ideas tend to flow more freely, and discussions can become more dynamic. These adjustments, though minor, offer a cumulative benefit to your physical and mental well-being.

Active commuting is another area ripe for enhancing your daily movement. Many people spend hours each week commuting, often sitting in cars or aboard public transport. By choosing to bike to work or walk part of the way, you engage your muscles, improve cardiovascular health, and reduce your reliance on motor vehicles. Biking, for instance, provides an excellent cardiovascular workout while minimizing environmental impact. Even if you live too far to bike the entire distance, consider parking further away and walking the remaining stretch. These choices contribute to your physical activity and provide an opportunity to clear your mind and enjoy your surroundings, turning a mundane task into a beneficial habit.

Creating an environment that encourages movement is crucial for promoting an active lifestyle. At work, consider using a standing desk, which can help reduce the amount of time you spend sitting and encourage more movement throughout the day. Standing while working can improve posture and increase alertness, keeping you engaged and productive. Additionally, incorporating active breaks into your day can revitalize your body and mind. Set reminders to stand up, stretch, or take a brief walk every hour. These breaks not only prevent prolonged periods of inactivity but also enhance focus and reduce stress. By fostering a culture that values movement, you're more likely to stay active and healthy in the long run.

These changes don't require a gym membership or special equipment; they simply involve a shift in mindset. By viewing every opportunity for movement as a chance to improve your health, you can transform your daily routine into a powerful tool for maintaining youthfulness and vitality. It's about embracing a lifestyle where activity is integrated seamlessly, not as an obligation, but as a natural expression of living well. This perspective not only supports your physical health but also encourages a more engaged and present way of life, where every step counts toward a healthier you.

MIND-BODY EXERCISES: YOGA AND TAI CHI FOR AGE REVERSAL

Incorporating mind-body exercises such as yoga and Tai Chi into your routine can be transformative, melding physical movement with mental focus to enhance overall well-being. These practices are not merely about stretching or slow movements; they represent a profound connection between the breath and body, creating a harmonious balance that promotes both physical health and mental clarity. As you flow through poses or sequences, the rhythmic breathing guides you, bringing awareness to the present moment and fostering a sense of inner peace. This integration of breath and movement is at the core of mind-body exercises, which offer a holistic approach to fitness that can dramatically impact your biological age.

Yoga and Tai Chi are particularly effective in supporting flexibility, balance, and stress reduction. Through regular practice, you improve proprioception, the body's ability to perceive its position in space, which enhances coordination and stability. This is crucial for preventing falls and maintaining independence as you age. Additionally, these exercises cultivate mental clarity, helping to clear the mind of clutter and distractions. The meditative nature of yoga and Tai Chi encourages a state of mindfulness, reducing stress and promoting relaxation. The benefits extend beyond the physical, offering a calming effect that can lead to improved emotional resilience and overall mental well-being.

For those new to these practices, starting with simple routines can ease the transition into a more mindful way of moving. Yoga's sun salutations provide an excellent introduction, combining basic poses with coordinated breathing to warm up the body and focus the mind. This sequence enhances flexibility and strength and establishes a rhythm that connects you to your breath. In Tai Chi, beginning with basic sequences allows you to explore the fluid movements that characterize this ancient martial art. These sequences are designed to promote balance and flow, making them accessible to individuals of all ages and fitness levels. Consistency in practice is key, and as you become more comfortable, you can gradually incorporate more advanced poses and sequences.

Mindfulness plays a pivotal role in maximizing the benefits of these exercises. By focusing on your breath during each pose, you deepen the connection between body and mind, enhancing the effectiveness of your practice. This focus helps to anchor you in the moment, allowing you to fully experience each movement and sensation. Meditation, often integrated into the routine, further enhances this mindfulness, encouraging introspection and self-awareness. Whether you practice in solitude or as part of a group, these moments of quiet reflection offer a sanctuary from the stresses of daily life, fostering a sense of calm and centeredness that extends beyond the mat or practice space.

Engaging in community participation can significantly enrich your experience with yoga and Tai Chi. Joining local classes or groups not only provides access to expert instruction but also fosters a sense of community and shared purpose. Yoga studios and Tai Chi parks offer environments where you can connect with others who share your interest in these practices, creating opportunities for support and encouragement. This communal aspect can motivate you to maintain a regular practice, while also introducing you to new perspectives and techniques. The social interaction inherent in group practice can enhance your enjoyment and commitment, making it more likely that you will continue to reap the benefits of these age-reversing exercises.

As you embrace these mind-body exercises, you may find that they become an integral part of your lifestyle, offering not just physical benefits but also a source of mental and emotional strength. The commitment to these practices can lead to profound changes in how you feel and function, supporting your goal of reversing biological age. This chapter has explored the physical and mental benefits of movement and exercise, and now we turn to the next crucial element in your age-reversal toolkit: cultivating healthy activities and relationships.

3

HABIT 3: CULTIVATING HEALTHY RELATIONSHIPS AND ACTIVITIES

Imagine a world where your friends and family are not just companions but vital contributors to your longevity and health. This concept isn't as far-fetched as it might seem. The strength of your social connections plays a critical role in determining not just how long you live, but how vibrant and fulfilling those years can be. Numerous studies have shown that individuals with robust social ties enjoy a lower risk of cardiovascular diseases and improved immune system function, a testament to the powerful influence of relationships on physical health. Social integration has been likened to other well-established health practices, offering protective benefits that help stave off illness and promote longevity. By fostering these connections, you are investing in a healthier, longer life.

Emotional support from loved ones is an indispensable component of health and wellness. Having people to turn to during challenging times reduces stress, which is detrimental to health if left unchecked. Social connections facilitate a decline in stress hormones, creating a buffer against the psychological strain that can accelerate aging. Moreover, these bonds enhance emotional resilience, equipping you to handle life's inevitable ups and downs more effectively. When you share your burdens, the load is lighter, and the path ahead is clearer. Emotional support is not just about being there for each other in times of need; it is about building a network of care that promotes mutual growth and strength.

Strengthening your social connections requires intentionality and effort but reaps immense rewards. Regular family gatherings are a simple yet profound way to nurture these bonds. Whether it's a weekly dinner, a shared hobby, or a holiday celebration, these moments reinforce the familial ties that serve as a foundation of support. Similarly, maintaining friendships through weekly phone calls can keep relationships vibrant and prevent the drift that often occurs with time and distance. These interactions don't need to be lengthy; rather, consistency is key, allowing for continual engagement and connection.

In our digital era, technology offers innovative ways to maintain and even enhance these bonds, provided it's used thoughtfully. Video calls have become an invaluable tool for staying in touch with distant loved ones, offering a sense of presence that transcends miles. Despite physical separation, seeing a familiar face and sharing a conversation in real-time can bridge the gap, maintaining and strengthening relational ties. Social media, too, can serve a positive role when utilized to connect with groups that share your interests. By joining online communities, you can find support, exchange ideas, and cultivate friendships that might not have been possible otherwise. However, it's essential to use these tools without letting them become a distraction, ensuring that digital interactions complement, rather than replace, face-to-face relationships.

Reflective Exercise: Mapping Your Social Web

Engage in this exercise to visualize and strengthen your social connections:

1. **Identify Your Circles**: List your closest family and friends. Consider how often you communicate and the depth of these relationships.
2. **Assess Your Engagement**: Reflect on how you connect with each person. Are there relationships that need more attention or revitalization?
3. **Set Connection Goals**: Establish realistic goals for improving these connections. This could be more frequent calls or planning get-togethers.
4. **Utilize Technology**: Identify digital tools that could enhance your interactions. Plan to use these tools to maintain regular contact without becoming reliant on them.

By understanding and actively nurturing your social connections, you can create a supportive network that enhances your emotional wellbeing and contributes significantly to your overall health and longevity.

COMMUNITY ENGAGEMENT: BUILDING A SUPPORT NETWORK

Community involvement is more than just participating in activities; it's about weaving yourself into the fabric of where you live. Being part of a community fosters a profound sense of belonging, which is essential for mental well-being. When you feel connected to those around you, it creates a foundation of support and shared resources that you can rely on. This network acts as a safety net, offering assistance and companionship in times of need. The relationships you build within your community can provide a buffer against life's challenges, enhancing your overall resilience and quality of life.

Engaging with your community can take many forms, each offering unique opportunities for connection and growth. Joining local clubs or organizations is a fantastic way to meet people who share similar interests or goals. Whether it's a book club, a gardening group, or a community sports team, these gatherings foster camaraderie and offer a chance to develop new skills. Participating in local events and fairs can also bring you closer to your neighbors. These events often celebrate the unique culture and spirit of your community, providing a platform for interaction and discovery. Through these activities, you not only become more integrated into your community but also contribute to its vibrancy and vitality.

Building a diverse social network is invaluable. Engaging with people from various backgrounds broadens your perspective and enhances your social skills. Exposure to different cultures, ideas, and life experiences enriches your understanding of the world, fostering empathy and adaptability. Such diversity can spark creativity and innovation, as you learn to see challenges from multiple angles. By cultivating relationships with a wide range of individuals, you create a tapestry of support that is both rich and resilient. This diversity strengthens your social web, equipping you to navigate the complexities of modern life with greater ease and confidence.

Support groups focused on health and wellness offer a unique platform for community engagement. These groups provide a space where individuals with shared goals can come together to offer encouragement, share experiences, and learn from one another. Fitness clubs, for example, not only promote physical health but also create a sense of camaraderie and motivation. Working out alongside others can make exercise more enjoyable and help you stay committed to your fitness goals. Similarly, mindfulness and meditation groups offer a sanctuary for mental rejuvenation, where participants can explore techniques to reduce stress and enhance well-being. These groups often foster a strong sense of community, as members support each other's journey toward improved health and happiness.

Interactive Element: Community Engagement Checklist

1. **Identify Your Interests**: Consider what activities or causes resonate with you. This could be anything from environmental conservation to arts and crafts.
2. **Research Local Opportunities**: Look for clubs, organizations, or events in your area that align with your interests. Libraries, community centers, and local websites are great resources.
3. **Reach Out and Participate**: Don't hesitate to attend meetings or events. Introduce yourself, share your interests, and be open to new experiences.
4. **Reflect on Your Experiences**: After engaging with your community, take time to reflect on what you enjoyed and what you learned. This can help you refine your involvement and deepen your connections.

By actively engaging with your community, you cultivate a network of support and shared purpose that enhances both your personal well-being and the collective health of your community.

PURPOSEFUL LIVING: FINDING PASSION AND FULFILLMENT

Living with purpose means more than just going through the motions of everyday life. It's about approaching each day with intention, clarity, and a sense of direction. Research has shown that individuals who cultivate a purposeful life experience increased life satisfaction and a significant reduction in depressive symptoms. When you wake up with a clear sense of what you want to accomplish and why, it sets a positive tone, influencing your mood and outlook. This mindset transforms challenges into opportunities for growth, fostering resilience and overall happiness. Purposeful living isn't just a philosophical concept; it's a practical approach to enhancing your quality of life.

Discovering what truly brings you joy is a pivotal step in living with purpose. Start by engaging in self-reflection to identify the activities that ignite your passion and excitement. Journaling can be an invaluable tool in this process. Take time to write about what energizes you, what you lose track of time doing, and what activities make you feel most alive. By exploring these insights, you can pinpoint your passions and begin to set goals that align with them. Setting goals is crucial as it provides direction and momentum, turning abstract desires into tangible pursuits. Whether it's learning a new skill, pursuing a creative hobby, or dedicating time to a cause you care about, aligning your actions with your passions infuses your life with meaning.

Purpose doesn't just enrich your daily experiences; it also has profound implications for cognitive health. Studies indicate that having a clear sense of purpose can enhance cognitive function, reducing the risk of dementia and improving memory and focus. Engaging with life purposefully stimulates brain activity, fostering cognitive resilience and delaying the onset of age-related cognitive decline. This link between purpose and cognitive health underscores the importance of staying mentally active and engaged. When you have something to strive for, your brain remains agile and adaptable, which is crucial for maintaining mental sharpness as you age.

Integrating purpose into your daily life involves more than just identifying your passions; it requires taking actionable steps to weave them into your routine. Volunteering for causes that resonate with you is an excellent way to channel your energy into meaningful endeavors. Not only does volunteering provide a sense of accomplishment, but it also connects you with like-minded individuals who share your values. This connection fosters a supportive environment where your contributions are valued and celebrated. Additionally, pursuing lifelong learning opportunities keeps your mind sharp and engaged. Whether through formal education or self-directed study, learning new things stimulates your brain, keeping it vibrant and healthy. By dedicating time to both volunteering and learning, you create a balanced life that reflects your deepest values and aspirations.

THE IMPACT OF VOLUNTEERING ON MENTAL AND PHYSICAL HEALTH

Volunteering is more than just an act of kindness; it is a profound means of enhancing both mental and physical health. Engaging in volunteer work fosters a deep sense of accomplishment, which can significantly uplift your mood. When you volunteer, you are not only contributing to the betterment of your community, but also investing in your own well-being. This involvement provides a unique opportunity to boost self-esteem, as you witness the tangible impact of your efforts. The satisfaction that comes from helping others can be a powerful antidote to feelings of inadequacy or low self-worth, replacing them with a sense of pride and purpose. Moreover, the positive emotions elicited from volunteering are infectious, often leading to an overall enhancement in mood and outlook on life. This positive shift in mental state can have lasting effects, contributing to a more optimistic and resilient mindset.

The physical health benefits of volunteering are equally noteworthy. Many volunteer activities inherently require physical movement, thereby increasing your activity levels without the monotony of a gym routine. Whether you're sorting donations at a local shelter, planting trees in an environmental clean-up project, or distributing meals at a food bank, these tasks engage your body in meaningful action. This increase in physical activity can help lower blood pressure and reduce stress, contributing to better cardiovascular health. The physical exertion involved in volunteering keeps the body active and stimulates the release of endorphins, which are natural mood enhancers. These chemical changes in the brain can lead to a reduction in stress and anxiety, making volunteering a holistic approach to health improvement. It's a win-win situation where you help others and enhance your own physical well-being.

Opportunities to volunteer are abundant and varied, allowing you to choose experiences that align with your interests and values. Local shelters and food banks are always in need of extra hands, providing an opportunity to assist those in immediate need. These environments offer a firsthand look at the impact of community efforts, making your contribution feel both significant and rewarding. For those passionate about the environment, participating in clean-up projects can be particularly fulfilling. These initiatives not only beautify public spaces, but also instill a sense of responsibility towards the planet. Volunteering in these settings offers a chance to connect with nature while actively contributing to its preservation. Exploring different volunteer opportunities allows you to discover new passions and skills, expanding your personal growth while making a difference.

Integrating volunteering into a busy schedule may seem challenging, but there are practical strategies to make it feasible. Micro-volunteering is a concept that has gained popularity for its flexibility and convenience. It involves small, manageable tasks that can be completed in short bursts of time, making it ideal for those with packed schedules. These tasks can range from writing letters to the elderly to helping with online research for a non-profit organization. Additionally, the rise of digital platforms has facilitated flexible online volunteering, allowing you to contribute from the comfort of your home. This can include tasks such as virtual tutoring, graphic design for charity organizations, or managing social media accounts for a cause you care about. By leveraging technology, you can engage in meaningful volunteer work without the constraints of traditional time commitments.

Balancing volunteering with other commitments requires thoughtful planning and prioritization. Start by assessing your current schedule and identifying pockets of time that can be dedicated to volunteer activities. Even a few hours a month can make a significant difference, both in the lives of those you help and in your own well-being. It's important to choose volunteer opportunities that resonate with you personally, as this alignment will enhance your motivation and commitment. Communicate your availability clearly with volunteer coordinators to ensure that your contributions fit seamlessly with your lifestyle. By consciously integrating volunteering into your routine, you can enjoy the myriad benefits it offers while maintaining balance in your personal and professional life.

HOBBIES THAT HEAL: CREATIVE OUTLETS FOR STRESS REDUCTION

In the hustle and bustle of daily life, finding a refuge through hobbies can be a powerful means to alleviate stress and rejuvenate the mind. Engaging in hobbies allows you to momentarily set aside life's pressures, offering a mental escape that refreshes and revitalizes. As you immerse yourself in an activity you love, your mind enters a state known as "flow," where time seems to vanish, and concerns fade into the background. This state of flow, characterized by deep focus and enjoyment, fosters mindfulness and reduces stress. Whether it's the rhythmic strokes of a paintbrush or the delicate touch needed to cultivate a garden, these moments of creativity can enhance your well-being by providing a sanctuary for your thoughts and emotions.

Certain hobbies stand out for their therapeutic effects, each offering unique benefits that support both mental and physical health. Painting, for instance, is a wonderful way to express emotions and calm the mind. The act of creating art allows you to explore your feelings without the need for words, providing a cathartic release that can soothe anxiety and promote relaxation. Gardening, on the other hand, connects you with nature, nurturing a sense of peace and fulfillment. Tending to plants requires patience and care, qualities that translate into a meditative practice as you cultivate life from the soil. This connection with nature offers a grounding experience, reminding you of the cycles of growth and renewal. Meanwhile, playing a musical instrument engages the mind in complex patterns of rhythm and melody, stimulating cognitive function and enhancing focus. Each note played or chord strummed becomes an exercise in mindfulness, keeping you present and engaged.

Beyond their personal benefits, hobbies also hold the potential to foster social connections, providing a shared space where like-minded individuals can gather. For example, joining a book club not only encourages you to explore new stories and ideas but also offers a platform for discussion and camaraderie. These gatherings create a sense of community, where members can share insights and perspectives, deepening their understanding of the material and each other. Similarly, participating in group art classes enables you to learn and grow in a collaborative environment. Working alongside fellow artists fosters a spirit of creativity and support, as you exchange techniques and inspire one another. These social interactions enrich your hobby experience, adding layers of enjoyment and fulfillment.

Finding the right hobby can be a journey of self-discovery, one that requires openness to exploration and experimentation. Start by trying out different activities to see what resonates with you. Attend workshops, join clubs, or simply experiment on your own to identify what sparks your interest. It's important to acknowledge that not every hobby will suit you, and that's perfectly okay. The goal is to find something that aligns with your personal interests and lifestyle, offering joy and satisfaction. Once you've identified a hobby that speaks to you, set aside dedicated time each week to engage in it. Whether it's an hour of painting on a Saturday morning or a few minutes of gardening each evening, consistency helps integrate the hobby into your routine, making it a cherished part of your life. Prioritizing this time nurtures your passion and provides a regular outlet for stress relief.

Incorporating hobbies into your life is not just about passing time; it's about enriching your existence with activities that bring joy, fulfillment, and peace. These creative outlets offer a unique blend of distraction and engagement, allowing you to step away from daily stressors and reconnect with yourself. By investing in hobbies, you cultivate a balanced lifestyle that supports mental and emotional health, fostering resilience and well-being. As you explore new interests and deepen existing ones, you'll discover that hobbies can heal, offering solace and happiness in a complex world.

DIGITAL DETOX: ENHANCING PRESENCE AND CONNECTION

In a world increasingly dominated by screens, the concept of a digital detox has become more important than ever. At its core, a digital detox involves taking deliberate breaks from technology, such as smartphones, tablets, and computers, to reclaim mental clarity and improve presence in our daily lives. Reducing screen time can lead to significant improvements in mental health, including a noticeable reduction in stress and anxiety. Constant notifications and the pressure to stay connected can leave you feeling overwhelmed, making it hard to focus on the present moment. By stepping away from screens, even if only for a short period each day, you allow your mind the space to breathe, reset, and refocus on what truly matters.

The negative impacts of excessive digital use are well-documented. Spending too much time in front of screens not only strains your eyes but also disrupts your natural sleep patterns. The blue light emitted by screens interferes with the production of melatonin, the hormone that regulates sleep, leading to difficulties falling and staying asleep. This can result in a cycle of sleep deprivation that affects your overall health and well-being. Moreover, the overuse of digital devices can lead to shallow social interactions, where screen-mediated communication replaces face-to-face conversations. This shift can diminish the quality of relationships, as digital interactions often lack the depth and nuance of real-life connections. The reduction in meaningful human contact can leave you feeling isolated, even when surrounded by people online.

Implementing a digital detox can be a liberating experience, freeing you from the constant pull of technology and allowing you to reconnect with the world around you. Start by scheduling designated tech-free times each day. This could be during meals, when you choose to focus on the flavors and company rather than scrolling through your phone. Alternatively, consider setting aside an hour before bed to unwind without screens, creating a calming evening routine that supports restful sleep. Another effective strategy is to establish device-free zones at home, such as the bedroom or dining area, where the focus is on relaxation and interaction rather than digital distractions. By creating these boundaries, you foster an environment that encourages presence and mindfulness.

The benefits of enhanced presence in your daily life are profound. When you are more present, you can engage more deeply with those around you, strengthening relationships and building stronger bonds. Conversations become richer, and you develop a greater appreciation for the subtleties of human interaction. This heightened awareness extends beyond personal relationships to include a deeper connection with your surroundings. You start to notice the beauty of a sunset, the sound of birds chirping, or the scent of fresh flowers. These moments, often overlooked in the rush of modern life, add depth and texture to your experience, enriching your sense of fulfillment and happiness. By choosing to be present, you invite more joy and meaning into your life, cultivating a sense of gratitude for the world around you. This chapter concludes with the understanding that nurturing presence through a digital detox can lead to a more connected and fulfilling life.

ADVOCATING FOR A HEALTHIER POPULATION

"It is health that is real wealth and not pieces of gold and silver."

— *MAHATMA GANDHI*

No matter how dubious you were about biological age reversal when we first started this journey, I'm pretty sure I caught your attention when I told you that by the time I was 72, I'd managed to reverse my biological age by 30 years. Few people don't want to know how to do this. With life expectancy increasing, most of us will have many years of retirement to look forward to, and we all want to be healthy enough to enjoy it as much as possible.

I'd even go a step further than this and suggest that it's something most of us want everyone to be able to do. We all want the people we care about to be the happiest and healthiest versions of themselves, and it's in all of our best interests to minimize the strain put on the healthcare system. The six core habits we're looking at throughout this book have the power to do that when more people adopt them, and because I know how well they work, I'm determined to help as many people as I can understand and implement them.

Now that we're halfway through our journey together and you're beginning to see what you can do to improve your own health and reverse your biological age, I'd like to invite you to join me on my mission to get this information to as many people as possible. All you need to do to make a big difference is leave a short review.

By leaving a review of this book on Amazon, you'll help more health-conscious readers find it and understand exactly what they can do to improve their health.

Scan the QR code below.

Reviews are how books find new readers, and those readers pass them on to more new readers. Before you know it, information is spreading like wildfire, and more people know exactly what they can do to reverse the effects of aging and make sure their health is in top shape.

Thank you so much for your support. I know it doesn't feel like much, but it does make a huge difference.

4

HABIT 4: MASTERING SLEEP FOR CELLULAR REGENERATION

Have you ever pondered why some mornings feel like you could conquer the world, while others leave you feeling drained before the day even begins? The secret often lies not in what you do during the day, but in how well you sleep at night. Sleep is not just a passive state of rest but a dynamic process that plays a crucial role in maintaining your body's health and vitality. Understanding the intricacies of sleep cycles can unlock profound benefits for cellular regeneration, enhancing your overall well-being and fortifying your body's defenses against the ravages of time.

UNDERSTANDING SLEEP CYCLES: THE FOUNDATION OF RESTORATIVE REST

Sleep is a complex tapestry woven from different stages, each serving unique functions essential for both body and mind. These stages cycle throughout the night, creating a pattern that is vital for restorative rest. The journey begins with the lighter stages of Non-Rapid Eye Movement (Non-REM) sleep. Stage 1 marks the transition between wakefulness and sleep, a phase where your body starts to relax, and your brain waves begin to slow down. As you drift deeper into Stage 2, your heart rate and breathing continue to decelerate, preparing your body for the deeper sleep to come. Stage 3, often referred to as deep sleep or slow-wave sleep, is where the magic of physical restoration occurs. During this time, your body repairs tissues, builds bone and muscle, and releases essential growth hormones. This stage is crucial for waking up refreshed and physically restored.

Then comes Rapid Eye Movement (REM) sleep, a fascinating stage where your brain becomes highly active. It is during this phase that dreaming occurs, and your eyes move rapidly beneath closed eyelids. REM sleep plays a critical role in memory processing and consolidation, as your brain takes the information gathered throughout the day and integrates it into long-term storage. It's like your brain's filing system, making sense of what you've learned and experienced, and helping you wake up with a clearer mind and better capacity for problem-solving. Without adequate REM sleep, your memory and cognitive functions can suffer, leading to difficulties in retaining new information and performing complex tasks.

Experiencing full sleep cycles, which last about 90 minutes and include all these stages, is paramount for optimal health. Each cycle builds upon the last, ensuring that both your body and brain receive the care they need. Skipping or shortening these cycles disrupts this delicate balance, increasing the risk of cognitive decline and impairing your ability to think clearly. Moreover, sleep cycles help regulate hormonal balance, which is vital for everything from mood stabilization to energy levels. When sleep cycles are consistently disrupted, it can lead to hormonal imbalances that affect your overall health, contributing to weight gain, mood swings, and even chronic conditions.

The consequences of disrupted sleep cycles extend beyond mere tiredness. Interrupted sleep can lead to an increased risk of metabolic disorders such as diabetes and obesity, as the body's ability to process glucose is impaired. Additionally, chronic sleep deprivation is linked to mood disturbances and irritability, affecting your relationships and productivity. Over time, the cumulative effects of poor sleep can take a toll on your physical and mental health, underscoring the importance of prioritizing quality sleep.

To maintain healthy sleep cycles, implementing practical strategies can make a world of difference. Establishing a consistent sleep schedule is one of the most effective ways to regulate your body's internal clock. Try to go to bed and wake up at the same time every day, even on weekends, to reinforce your natural sleep-wake rhythm. This consistency helps your body anticipate sleep, making it easier to fall asleep and stay asleep. Additionally, limiting exposure to screens before bed is crucial, as the blue light emitted by devices can interfere with your body's production of melatonin, the hormone that regulates sleep. Aim to power down electronic devices at least an hour before bedtime, allowing your body to unwind and prepare for restful sleep. By understanding and respecting the complexities of your sleep cycles, you can enhance your body's ability to regenerate and rejuvenate.

Interactive Element: Sleep Cycle Reflection

Reflect on your current sleep habits with these prompts to enhance your understanding and improve your sleep quality:

1. **Track Your Sleep**: Keep a sleep diary for a week, noting when you go to bed, when you wake up, and how rested you feel. Look for patterns and areas for improvement.

2. **Evaluate Screen Time**: Reflect on your evening screen habits. Are there opportunities to reduce screen time before bed to improve sleep quality?
3. **Identify Disruptions**: Consider factors that commonly disrupt your sleep. It could be noise, stress, or irregular bedtimes. What can you change to address these issues?
4. **Set a Sleep Goal**: Based on your reflections, set a goal for improving your sleep habits. This could be establishing a consistent bedtime or reducing screen exposure before sleep.

By taking the time to understand your sleep cycles and make informed adjustments, you can create a foundation for restorative rest and better health.

CREATING A SLEEP SANCTUARY: OPTIMIZING YOUR ENVIRONMENT

Imagine walking into a room where the world seems to pause, inviting you to leave behind the day's chaos and embrace tranquility. This is the essence of a sleep sanctuary—a place meticulously crafted to enhance the quality of your rest. A well-designed sleep environment is pivotal for achieving restorative sleep, a cornerstone of rejuvenation. Begin with the basics: the room should be dark and quiet. Darkness signals your body to produce melatonin, the hormone that regulates sleep. Use blackout curtains to block out disruptive light, even the faint glow of streetlights. Silence is equally crucial, as noise can jolt you out of precious deep sleep. If absolute silence isn't feasible, a white noise machine can mask disturbances, helping maintain the peace needed for uninterrupted rest.

Your bed should be a haven of comfort, supporting your body in all the right places. Invest in quality bedding, which includes a supportive mattress and pillows that cater to your sleep position. A medium-firm mattress generally strikes the right balance for most sleepers, promoting spinal alignment and reducing pressure points. Pillows should cradle your neck, maintaining its natural curve to prevent stiffness. Choose breathable sheets that keep you comfortable throughout the night, ensuring you wake up refreshed. Remember, your bed is more than a piece of furniture; it's an investment in your health and well-being.

Consider the room's temperature and lighting, two factors that significantly influence sleep onset and quality. A cool room, ideally between 60 and 67 degrees Fahrenheit, can promote deeper sleep by lowering your core body temperature. This cooling effect helps signal to your body that it's time to rest. Adjust your thermostat accordingly, or use fans to maintain this optimal range. Lighting plays a pivotal role too. Harsh lights can disrupt your internal clock, so dim the lights as bedtime approaches to mimic the natural transition from day to night. If needed, use blackout curtains to eliminate any residual light, aiding in a more profound and uninterrupted sleep.

Aromatherapy can enhance your sleep sanctuary, with scents that soothe and relax. Lavender essential oil is renowned for its calming effects, often used to reduce anxiety and promote restful sleep. A few drops on your pillow or a diffuser can fill the room with its tranquil aroma, setting the stage for a peaceful night. Chamomile, another sleep-promoting scent, can be used in a similar manner, offering a gentle, soothing fragrance that eases tension. These natural remedies harness the power of scent to create a calming environment, preparing your mind and body for the restorative sleep ahead.

Minimizing disruptions is key to maintaining a serene sleep environment. Removing electronic devices from your bedroom can have a profound impact, as screens emit blue light that can interfere with your sleep cycle. Create a tech-free zone, allowing your bedroom to become a place solely dedicated to rest and relaxation. If external noises are an issue, consider utilizing earplugs or a white noise machine to block out disturbances. The gentle hum of white noise can mask sudden sounds, preventing them from interrupting your sleep. By addressing these potential disruptions, you craft a space that supports a seamless transition into restful slumber.

EVENING RITUALS: PREPARING YOUR MIND AND BODY FOR SLEEP

As the day winds down, establishing evening rituals can be a powerful way to signal to your body that it's time to transition to rest. These rituals aren't just about routine; they're about creating a serene prelude to sleep, helping to reduce stress and prepare both your mind and body for a restorative night. Consistency in bedtime habits is key. By adhering to a regular routine, you train your body to anticipate sleep, making it easier to drift off when your head hits the pillow. This consistency can be as simple as following the same sequence of activities each night, such as brushing your teeth, dimming the lights, and slipping into your favorite pajamas. These small, habitual actions cue your brain to begin winding down, setting the stage for sleep.

Incorporating calming activities into your nightly routine can further enhance your sleep preparation. Consider setting aside time to read a book—one made of paper, not pixels. The tactile experience of turning pages can be soothing, allowing you to escape into a story without the disruptive blue light of screens.

Alternatively, gentle yoga or stretching exercises can help relax tense muscles and quiet a busy mind. These movements encourage the release of tension accumulated throughout the day, promoting physical relaxation that complements mental calmness. The key is to choose activities that you find enjoyable and relaxing, making them a cherished part of your evening ritual.

Mindfulness techniques can play a crucial role in transitioning to sleep, helping to clear your mind of the day's clutter and focus on the present moment. Guided meditation sessions, whether through an app or a simple practice of focusing on your breath, can center your thoughts and ease mental chatter. Meditation encourages relaxation by activating the body's parasympathetic nervous system, which helps slow your heart rate and reduce stress hormones. Deep breathing exercises, like inhaling slowly through your nose and exhaling through your mouth, can also be effective. This practice calms your mind and physically prepares your body for sleep by promoting relaxation and reducing tension.

A digital detox before bed can significantly improve your sleep onset and quality. The blue light emitted by screens can interfere with your natural sleep-wake cycle, making it harder to fall asleep when you finally turn off your devices. Establishing a digital curfew, where you power down electronics at least an hour before bed, can help mitigate this effect. Use this time to engage in analog activities that promote relaxation and reflection. Journaling, for example, provides a creative outlet to express thoughts and feelings, helping to free your mind from lingering worries. Writing about your day or jotting down things you're grateful for can create a sense of closure, allowing you to enter sleep with a calm and settled mind.

THE ROLE OF CIRCADIAN RHYTHMS IN BIOLOGICAL AGE REVERSAL

Imagine your body as a finely tuned orchestra, with each organ playing its part in harmony with the others. This synchronization is largely governed by circadian rhythms, our internal clocks that align bodily functions with the 24-hour day-night cycle. These rhythms dictate the ebb and flow of various biological processes, influencing everything from sleep-wake patterns to hormone release. At the heart of this system lies the suprachiasmatic nucleus (SCN), a cluster of neurons in the brain that acts as a master clock, orchestrating these rhythms by responding to light cues. When you expose yourself to natural light in the morning, you help set this clock, reinforcing the natural cycle of alertness and restfulness. This synchronization ensures that energy levels peak during the day and decline at night, facilitating a balanced and efficient daily routine.

Circadian rhythms play a critical role in aging, impacting cellular repair processes and metabolic functions. When these rhythms are aligned with natural cycles, your body can efficiently repair damaged cells, maintain metabolic homeostasis, and regulate energy expenditure. This alignment supports the body's ability to rejuvenate during sleep, which is vital for reversing biological age. A well-synced circadian rhythm enhances your body's natural antioxidant production, reducing oxidative stress and slowing down the aging process. Furthermore, it optimizes the function of mitochondria, the energy powerhouses of your cells, ensuring that energy production remains high and efficient as you age. This optimization is crucial for sustaining youthful vitality and preventing the decline in metabolic function that often accompanies aging.

Aligning your daily activities with natural circadian rhythms can significantly enhance your health and longevity. Begin by prioritizing exposure to natural light, especially in the morning. This simple act can reinforce your body's internal clock, promoting a healthier sleep-wake cycle. Consistent meal timing is another effective strategy. By eating meals at the same times each day, you help stabilize your body's metabolic processes and support digestive health. This consistency aids in regulating insulin levels, reducing the risk of metabolic disorders. Additionally, engaging in regular physical activity during daylight hours can further synchronize your body's rhythms, enhancing overall health and well-being.

When circadian rhythms fall out of sync, the consequences can be far-reaching, affecting both physical and mental health. Disrupted rhythms can lead to elevated levels of stress hormones like cortisol, which, in excess, can wreak havoc on your body's systems. High cortisol levels are linked to increased risk of chronic conditions such as cardiovascular disease, obesity, and type 2 diabetes. Moreover, circadian misalignment can compromise your immune system, leaving you more susceptible to infections and illnesses. This disruption also impairs cognitive function, leading to difficulties in concentration and memory retention. Over time, the cumulative effects of disrupted circadian rhythms can accelerate biological aging, underscoring the importance of maintaining alignment with natural cycles.

NUTRIENTS AND SUPPLEMENTS FOR QUALITY SLEEP

Quality sleep is not merely about the hours spent in bed, but the restfulness and restoration achieved during that time. A crucial component of this rejuvenation process lies in the nutrients your body receives. Magnesium, for instance, plays a pivotal role in sleep by promoting muscle relaxation. This essential mineral helps to calm the nervous system, easing tension that can interfere with restful slumber. It acts by binding to GABA receptors in the brain, reducing nerve activity and facilitating relaxation. Foods rich in magnesium, such as leafy greens, nuts, and seeds, can enhance your diet and support better sleep. Almonds and walnuts, in particular, are excellent sources, offering a convenient snack option that contributes to your overall magnesium intake. By including these foods in your diet, you support not just muscle relaxation but also the broader benefits of magnesium, which include bone health and energy production.

Tryptophan is another key nutrient that significantly impacts sleep quality. This amino acid serves as a precursor to serotonin, a neurotransmitter that regulates mood and sleep cycles. Serotonin is further converted into melatonin, the hormone responsible for sleep regulation. Foods high in tryptophan, such as turkey and bananas, can support this biochemical pathway, enhancing the body's ability to produce serotonin and, subsequently, melatonin. Incorporating these foods into your evening meal can effectively prime your body for a peaceful night's rest. Turkey, often associated with post-Thanksgiving drowsiness, is a particularly potent source, while bananas offer a dual benefit with their magnesium content. By consuming tryptophan-rich foods, you not only support sleep but also improve mood regulation and emotional wellbeing.

Beyond natural nutrients, certain supplements can be beneficial in promoting restful sleep. Melatonin is perhaps the most well-known of these, often used to regulate sleep cycles, especially in cases of jet lag or shift work. This supplement mimics the natural hormone, helping to reset your internal clock when it's disrupted. Taking melatonin in the evening can signal to your body that it's time to wind down, making it easier to fall asleep. However, it's important to use it judiciously, as long-term reliance can interfere with the body's natural production. Valerian root is another supplement known for its anxiolytic properties, reducing anxiety that can prevent you from drifting off to sleep. While it may not work for everyone, many find that it helps ease nervous tension, allowing for a more natural transition into slumber. Combining these supplements with a balanced diet can optimize your sleep quality, providing both immediate benefits and supporting long-term health.

Dietary choices play a fundamental role in sleep health, and careful consideration can make a significant difference. Incorporating foods rich in magnesium and tryptophan is a step in the right direction, but overall dietary habits are equally important. Avoiding caffeine in the afternoon and evening is crucial, as it can linger in your system for hours, disrupting your ability to fall asleep. Opt for herbal teas or water instead, allowing your body to relax as bedtime approaches. Similarly, heavy meals before bed can interfere with sleep, as your body diverts energy to digestion rather than rest and repair. Aim for lighter, easily digestible meals in the evening, such as salads or soups, which satisfy hunger without burdening your system. These dietary adjustments, while simple, can have profound effects on your sleep quality, supporting a more tranquil and rejuvenating night's rest.

Balanced nutrition is not just about individual foods or supplements; it's about creating a harmonious dietary pattern that supports all aspects of health, including sleep. By focusing on nutrient-rich foods and mindful eating habits, you create a foundation for better sleep and overall wellbeing. This approach reinforces the body's natural rhythms, enhancing your ability to fall asleep and stay asleep. It's a holistic strategy that empowers you to take control of your sleep health, improving not just the quality of your rest but also your energy levels, mood, and resilience during waking hours. Embracing these principles can transform your nights, leading to more vibrant and productive days.

OVERCOMING INSOMNIA: PRACTICAL SOLUTIONS FOR BETTER SLEEP

Insomnia, a common yet often misunderstood condition, can manifest in several forms, each affecting your sleep differently. Short-term insomnia, typically lasting a few days to a few weeks, is often triggered by stress or a change in schedule, such as jet lag or a new job. This type of insomnia, though temporary, can disrupt your nightly rest and lead to daytime fatigue. On the other hand, chronic insomnia is a more persistent problem, occurring at least three times a week for three months or longer. This prolonged struggle with sleep impairs daily functioning and increases the risk of various health issues, from anxiety to heart disease. Understanding these distinctions is essential, as they guide the strategies used to address the underlying causes and improve sleep quality over time.

Stress and anxiety are primary culprits in the development of insomnia. When your mind is racing with worries or your body is tense with stress, falling asleep can seem impossible. These emotional states heighten arousal and make it difficult for your mind to shut down, leading to restless nights. Poor sleep hygiene, the collection of habits that influence sleep quality, also plays a significant role. Irregular sleep schedules, excessive caffeine consumption, and stimulating activities before bed can all interfere with your ability to fall and stay asleep. Recognizing and addressing these factors is crucial in overcoming insomnia and regaining restful sleep.

Fortunately, several evidence-based solutions can help combat insomnia and restore your sleep quality. Cognitive Behavioral

Therapy for Insomnia (CBT-I) is one of the most effective treatments, focusing on changing the thoughts and behaviors that contribute to sleep problems. Through CBT-I, you learn to challenge unhelpful beliefs about sleep and develop healthier sleep habits. This therapy can involve techniques such as stimulus control, which trains your brain to associate the bed with sleep rather than wakefulness, and sleep hygiene education, which emphasizes the importance of a regular sleep schedule and a conducive sleep environment. Another method, sleep restriction therapy, limits the time spent in bed to increase sleep efficiency. By initially reducing the time allowed for sleep, this approach builds a stronger sleep drive, eventually leading to longer and more restful nights.

In addition to these therapeutic techniques, lifestyle changes can significantly enhance sleep quality. Regular physical activity is a powerful ally in promoting better sleep, as it helps to reduce stress and regulate your body's internal clock. Engaging in exercise during the day, even if it's just a brisk walk, can make it easier to fall asleep at night and improve sleep depth. Mindfulness practices, such as meditation and yoga, offer another layer of support by calming the mind and reducing anxiety. These practices encourage relaxation and present-moment awareness, helping you to release the tensions of the day and prepare for sleep. By integrating these activities into your routine, you create a supportive environment that facilitates better rest.

To effectively tackle insomnia, it's important to consider both immediate interventions and long-term lifestyle adjustments. Short-term solutions, such as CBT-I and sleep restriction therapy, provide tools to address current sleep difficulties and can yield noticeable improvements within weeks. However, sustaining these benefits requires ongoing commitment to healthy habits and stress management techniques. Cultivating a lifestyle that prioritizes physical activity, mindfulness, and consistent sleep schedules can help maintain sleep improvements and prevent future disruptions. This holistic approach enhances sleep quality and supports overall well-being, reinforcing the connection between restful nights and vibrant days.

Through understanding insomnia's complexities and implementing targeted strategies, you can transform your sleep experience and reclaim the restorative rest your body craves. As you move forward, consider how these insights can be applied to other areas of health and wellness, recognizing the interconnectedness of sleep with broader aspects of life. The next chapter will delve into the crucial role of stress management in maintaining balance and promoting longevity, building upon the foundation of restful sleep established here.

5

HABIT 5: MANAGING STRESS FOR LONGEVITY

Consider this: when was the last time you truly felt at ease, without the constant buzz of stress nudging at the edges of your consciousness? In our modern world, stress has become an all-too-familiar companion, often lurking in the shadows of our daily routines. Yet, its impact on our health is profound and far-reaching. Understanding the biology of stress and its role in accelerating aging is crucial if we are to harness its effects and prolong our vitality. Stress isn't just a mental game; it's a complex physiological process that can alter how we age, affecting everything from our cellular health to our overall longevity.

At the heart of our stress response lies the hypothalamic-pituitary-adrenal (HPA) axis, a network that orchestrates the body's reaction to stressors. When you encounter a perceived threat, whether physical or emotional, your brain activates this axis, setting off a cascade of hormonal signals. The hypothalamus releases corticotropin-releasing hormone (CRH), prompting the pituitary gland to secrete adrenocorticotropic hormone (ACTH). This hormone travels through your bloodstream to the adrenal glands, nestled atop your kidneys, triggering them to release stress hormones such as cortisol and adrenaline. These hormones prepare your body for a "fight or flight" response, increasing heart rate and energy availability, sharpening focus, and heightening awareness. This response, while evolutionarily designed to protect us, can become detrimental when persistently activated, leading to chronic stress and its associated health impacts.

Chronic stress, a state where your body's stress response is continuously engaged, can wreak havoc on your health and accelerate aging. One of the most significant effects of prolonged stress is its impact on telomeres, the protective caps at the ends of chromosomes that shorten each time a cell divides. Research has shown that chronic stress can accelerate telomere shortening, hastening cellular aging and increasing susceptibility to age-related diseases. Furthermore, stress elevates oxidative stress levels, an imbalance between free radicals and antioxidants in the body, which can damage cells, proteins, and DNA, further exacerbating the aging process. The continuous strain on your body also affects your immune system, leaving you more vulnerable to infections and chronic illnesses.

The concept of allostatic load provides a framework for understanding how cumulative stress impacts the body's ability to adapt and maintain stability. Allostasis refers to the process by which your body achieves stability through change, involving the interplay of the neuroendocrine, autonomic, and immune systems. However, when faced with chronic stress, your body's adaptive mechanisms can become overwhelmed, leading to an allostatic load, or the wear and tear on the body that accumulates over time. This burden can manifest in various ways, including hypertension, reduced anabolic processes, and even brain atrophy. The immune system, too, suffers under the weight of allostatic load, resulting in impaired function and increased inflammation, which are precursors to several age-related diseases.

Recognizing the signs of stress in your body is crucial for managing its effects and mitigating its impact on aging. Physical indicators such as muscle tension and headaches are common, often manifesting as tightness in the neck, shoulders, and back, or as persistent headaches that seem to have no clear cause. These symptoms are your body's way of signaling that it's under duress. On an emotional level, stress can lead to mood swings, where you experience sudden shifts in emotions, ranging from irritability and anger to sadness and anxiety. You might also notice changes in sleep patterns, with difficulty falling or staying asleep, or waking up feeling unrested. Anxiety, a state of heightened apprehension and worry, often accompanies chronic stress, further exacerbating its physical symptoms and creating a vicious cycle that can be challenging to break.

Interactive Element: Stress Awareness Checklist

- **Physical Signs:** Note any frequent headaches, muscle tension, fatigue, or digestive issues.
- **Emotional Indicators:** Reflect on mood swings, anxiety, irritability, or feelings of being overwhelmed.
- **Behavioral Changes:** Observe any changes in sleep patterns, eating habits, or withdrawal from social activities.

By becoming attuned to these signals, you can take proactive steps to manage stress more effectively, which is essential for maintaining your health and longevity.

MINDFULNESS AND MEDITATION: TOOLS FOR STRESS REDUCTION

Imagine a practice that allows you to step away from the chaos of everyday life, grounding you in the present moment and offering clarity amidst the noise. This is the essence of mindfulness and meditation. At its core, mindfulness is about present moment awareness—being fully engaged with what you're doing, with a gentle acceptance of your thoughts and feelings. It encourages non-judgmental observation, allowing you to witness your experiences without getting caught up in them. Meditation, a practice rooted in mindfulness, trains your mind to focus and redirect thoughts, promoting emotional stability and peace. Together, these practices serve as a balm for the stress that so often accompanies modern living, offering a sanctuary of calm and resilience.

The benefits of regular mindfulness and meditation practice extend far beyond momentary relaxation. Engaging consistently with these practices can lead to a marked reduction in anxiety and depression, as they allow you to break free from the cyclical nature of these states by fostering a more balanced outlook. Emotional regulation improves as you learn to respond to situations with awareness rather than react impulsively. This shift can lead to more harmonious relationships and a more profound understanding of yourself. Physically, meditation has been shown to lower blood pressure, reduce chronic pain, and even strengthen the immune system. These benefits collectively contribute to a healthier, more balanced lifestyle, making mindfulness and meditation invaluable tools in managing stress and enhancing longevity.

For those new to meditation, starting with simple techniques can make the practice feel accessible and rewarding. One such method is the body scan meditation, where you focus your attention on different parts of your body, from head to toe, noting any sensations without judgment. This practice can help you become more attuned to your physical state, promoting relaxation and awareness. Another technique is loving-kindness meditation, which involves generating feelings of compassion and love for yourself and others. This practice fosters a sense of connection and empathy, counteracting feelings of isolation or negativity. Both methods require only a few minutes a day and can be tailored to fit your schedule, making them easy to incorporate into your routine.

Incorporating mindfulness into daily life doesn't necessarily require setting aside large blocks of time. Instead, it can be woven into the fabric of everyday activities, transforming mundane moments into opportunities for mindfulness. Mindful eating, for example, encourages you to savor each bite, focusing on the flavors, textures, and aromas of your food. This practice not only enhances your dining experience but also promotes healthier eating habits by allowing you to recognize hunger and satiety cues. Similarly, walking meditation invites you to be present with each step, feeling the ground beneath your feet and observing your surroundings with curiosity and openness. Taking a mindful walk in nature can be especially rejuvenating, as it combines the calming effects of mindfulness with the restorative power of the natural world.

Reflection Exercise: Daily Mindfulness Integration

- **Mindful Morning:** Spend the first five minutes of your day in silence, focusing on your breathing and setting a positive intention for the day.
- **Midday Pause:** During lunch, practice mindful eating by chewing slowly and appreciating each flavor.

- **Evening Reflection:** Before bed, journal briefly about your day, noting moments of mindfulness and gratitude.

Through these simple yet profound practices, you can cultivate a deeper sense of peace and resilience, equipping yourself to handle stress with grace and equanimity.

BREATHING TECHNIQUES: HARNESSING THE POWER OF BREATH

Breathing, a fundamental yet often overlooked function, holds incredible power over our physiological state, particularly in relation to stress. The way you breathe can significantly influence how your body responds to stressors. At its core, breathing activates the parasympathetic nervous system, the branch of your nervous system responsible for promoting a state of relaxation and calm. When you engage in deep, controlled breathing, your body shifts from the stress-induced "fight or flight" mode to "rest and digest." This transition not only reduces heart rate and lowers blood pressure but also fosters a sense of tranquility that counteracts the chaos of stress. By consciously altering your breathing patterns, you can tap into this natural mechanism to manage stress effectively.

One of the simplest yet most effective techniques for stress reduction is diaphragmatic breathing, often referred to as "belly breathing." This method involves inhaling deeply through the nose, allowing your diaphragm to expand and your abdomen to rise. As you exhale slowly through your mouth, your belly falls, completing the breath cycle. This type of breathing encourages full oxygen exchange, slowing down the heartbeat, and stabilizing blood pressure. Another technique, box breathing, is popular among athletes and military personnel for its ability to enhance focus and calmness. It involves inhaling for four counts, holding the breath for four counts, exhaling for four counts, and holding again for four counts. This rhythmic breathing pattern helps regulate your nervous system, providing immediate stress relief. Alternate nostril breathing, a practice rooted in yogic traditions, balances the left and right hemispheres of the brain, promoting mental clarity and emotional stability. By alternating the nostril you breathe through, you can harmonize your energy and reduce anxiety.

The benefits of incorporating regular breathing exercises into your routine are both immediate and long-lasting. On a short-term basis, these exercises enhance focus and concentration, allowing you to approach tasks with a clear and centered mind. They also provide a quick and effective way to decrease stress-related symptoms, such as tension, restlessness, and even physical discomfort. Over time, consistent practice of breathing techniques can lead to improved emotional regulation, heightened resilience to stress, and a more balanced emotional state. The cumulative effect of these exercises supports overall mental health, creating a stable foundation for facing life's challenges with confidence and grace.

Integrating breathing exercises into your daily schedule doesn't require a major time commitment and can be seamlessly woven into your existing routine. Start your day with a morning breathing routine to set a calm and focused tone. Spend just five minutes practicing diaphragmatic breathing before you get out of bed, allowing your body to transition gently from sleep to wakefulness. During the workday, take short breathing breaks to recharge and refocus. Whether you're at your desk or stepping outside for fresh air, dedicate a few minutes to practicing box breathing or alternate nostril breathing. These breaks enhance productivity and prevent stress from building up throughout the day. In the evening, incorporate a calming breathing exercise into your bedtime routine. This not only prepares your mind and body for restful sleep but also helps release the accumulated stress of the day. By embracing these simple yet powerful techniques, you can cultivate a sense of peace and resilience that permeates every aspect of your life.

COGNITIVE BEHAVIORAL STRATEGIES FOR STRESS MANAGEMENT

Imagine being able to shift your mindset from one of stress and overwhelm to calm and control. This is the promise of cognitive behavioral therapy (CBT), a widely used approach in psychology that helps individuals identify and change negative thought patterns that contribute to stress and anxiety. At its core, CBT is based on the idea that our thoughts, feelings, and behaviors are interconnected. By restructuring negative thought patterns and developing coping strategies, you can alter your emotional responses and behaviors in a meaningful way. CBT empowers you to take control of your mental landscape, offering a path to reduce stress and enhance your overall well-being. It's about understanding that while you may not always have control over the situations you face, you do have control over how you perceive and react to them.

The effectiveness of CBT in managing stress and anxiety is well-documented, with numerous studies supporting its use as a powerful tool for mental health. Research has shown that CBT not only helps reduce symptoms of stress and anxiety but also improves mental resilience, enabling individuals to cope more effectively with life's challenges. This form of therapy equips you with practical skills to manage stress-induced behaviors, such as avoidance or rumination, that often exacerbate anxiety. By providing a structured framework for understanding and addressing the cognitive distortions that underlie stress, CBT fosters a greater sense of control and empowerment. It teaches you to replace unhelpful thought patterns with more balanced, realistic perspectives, leading to a healthier, more adaptive way of thinking.

To put CBT into practice, consider engaging in thought record keeping, a technique that involves monitoring your thoughts and identifying patterns that contribute to stress. This exercise encourages you to challenge these thoughts, asking yourself whether they are based on facts or assumptions. By questioning the validity of these thoughts, you can begin to replace them with more rational, balanced beliefs. Behavioral experiments are another practical tool within CBT, allowing you to test the accuracy of your negative beliefs by experimenting with new behaviors and observing the outcomes. This hands-on approach helps you gather evidence that contradicts your fears or assumptions, fostering a more positive outlook.

Journaling is a complementary practice that enhances the effectiveness of CBT by providing a space for reflection and cognitive restructuring. Gratitude journaling, for example, involves regularly writing down things you are thankful for, which can shift your focus away from stressors and towards positive aspects of your life. This practice has been shown to improve mood and increase feelings of well-being by promoting a more appreciative mindset. Reflective writing exercises, on the other hand, allow you to explore your thoughts and emotions in depth, facilitating greater self-awareness and insight. By writing about stressful experiences, you can gain clarity on the underlying issues and develop strategies for coping more effectively.

Reflection Section: Journaling Prompts for Stress Management

- **Identify Stress Triggers:** Write about a recent situation that caused you stress. What thoughts and emotions did it trigger, and how did you respond?
- **Challenge Negative Thoughts:** Reflect on a negative thought pattern you've noticed. How can you reframe it more positively or realistically?
- **Explore Gratitude:** List three things you are grateful for today. How do these aspects of your life bring you joy or peace?

These CBT techniques and journaling practices offer a structured approach to managing stress, empowering you to take charge of your mental landscape and cultivate resilience.

THE EFFECTS OF NATURE ON STRESS AND LONGEVITY

Imagine stepping into a forest where sunlight filters through the leaves, casting dappled shadows on the ground. The air is rich with the scent of pine, and the gentle rustle of leaves provides a soothing background symphony. This isn't just a picturesque scene; it's a form of therapy known as forest bathing, or Shinrin-yoku. Originating in Japan, this practice involves immersing oneself in the natural environment, allowing the sights, sounds, and smells of the forest to wash over you. It's a deliberate act of connecting with nature, which has been shown to reduce stress and enhance overall health. The benefits of spending time in green spaces extend beyond mere relaxation. They facilitate a profound physiological response that can lower cortisol levels and promote a sense of well-being.

The science behind nature's impact on stress is compelling. Numerous studies have documented how exposure to natural environments can significantly reduce cortisol, the body's primary stress hormone. In one study, participants who engaged in forest bathing experienced a marked decrease in cortisol levels compared to those who remained in urban settings. This reduction in stress hormones translates to lower blood pressure and heart rate, creating a state of calm that enhances both mental clarity and mood. Furthermore, being in nature stimulates the production of serotonin, a neurotransmitter associated with feelings of happiness and well-being. This natural boost to your mood fosters mental clarity, allowing you to think more clearly and make better decisions. The therapeutic effects of nature alleviate stress and support cognitive function, providing a holistic approach to managing life's challenges.

Incorporating outdoor activities that combine physical movement with nature exposure can amplify these benefits. Hiking, for example, offers a perfect blend of cardiovascular exercise and nature immersion. The rhythmic motion of walking, combined with the ever-changing scenery, promotes mindfulness and keeps your focus on the present moment. As you hike through natural settings, your body releases endorphins, enhancing your mood and counteracting stress. Gardening is another activity that fosters relaxation and connection with nature. The act of tending to plants, feeling the soil between your fingers, and witnessing the growth of life provides a sense of accomplishment and peace. Both hiking and gardening encourage you to slow down, appreciate the beauty around you, and engage in a form of active meditation that nourishes the mind and body.

If stepping outside isn't always feasible, you can create a nature-inspired haven within your home. Incorporating elements of nature into your living space can have a significant impact on stress reduction and overall well-being. One simple yet effective way to invite nature indoors is by adding houseplants. These green companions enhance air quality by filtering toxins and provide a visual reminder of the natural world. The presence of plants has been shown to reduce stress and promote a sense of calm, transforming your home into a sanctuary of tranquility. Additionally, ensuring ample natural light exposure can uplift your mood and regulate your circadian rhythms, which play a crucial role in sleep and overall health. Position your workspace near a window or use light-filtering curtains to make the most of daylight.

Creating a nature-inspired space doesn't require a complete home renovation. Small changes can make a significant difference in how you feel. Consider arranging furniture to maximize views of outdoor landscapes or adding nature-themed artwork that reflects the serenity of the natural world. Water features, such as tabletop fountains, can introduce the soothing sounds of flowing water, further enhancing your connection with nature. These elements enhance your living environment and provide a retreat from the busyness of life. By surrounding yourself with natural beauty, you invite a sense of peace and harmony into your daily routine, supporting your journey towards stress reduction and longevity.

BUILDING RESILIENCE: THRIVING AMIDST LIFE'S CHALLENGES

Resilience is a powerful trait that enables individuals to adapt to adversity and emerge stronger. It's not just about bouncing back from setbacks; it's about growing through them. The ability to navigate life's challenges without succumbing to stress is crucial for maintaining mental and physical health, especially as we age. Resilient people possess a mental fortitude that allows them to withstand the pressures of life, maintaining a sense of calm and control in the face of uncertainty. This strength is cultivated through experience, but it's also something you can consciously develop, enhancing your capacity to manage stress and protect against the wear and tear of aging.

Take a moment to consider the traits that characterize resilient individuals. Optimism is often at the forefront, as it fuels a positive outlook that sees opportunities rather than obstacles. Optimistic people tend to view challenges as temporary and surmountable, which gives them the courage to persevere. Alongside optimism, the capacity for emotional regulation is key. This involves managing emotions effectively, so they don't become overwhelming or dictate your actions. Resilient individuals can acknowledge their feelings without letting them take control, allowing for thoughtful responses rather than impulsive reactions. This emotional intelligence is a cornerstone of resilience, promoting stability and reducing the impact of stress on both mind and body.

Building resilience requires intentional strategies that can be woven into everyday life. Developing a growth mindset is one such approach, encouraging you to view challenges as opportunities for learning and development. This mindset fosters a love for lifelong learning and a willingness to embrace new experiences, seeing failures as valuable lessons rather than setbacks. Cultivating strong social connections is equally important, as relationships provide support and encouragement during difficult times. Surrounding yourself with positive, like-minded individuals can bolster your resilience, offering different perspectives and solutions. Whether through family, friends, or community groups, these connections form a safety net that helps you weather life's storms.

Self-care practices play a pivotal role in maintaining resilience and should not be overlooked. Prioritizing rest and relaxation is essential for replenishing your energy reserves and preventing burnout. This could involve setting aside time each day for activities that bring you joy, whether it's reading a book, taking a leisurely walk, or indulging in a creative hobby. By engaging in activities that fulfill you, you nurture your spirit and build resilience against stress. Restful sleep, regular exercise, and balanced nutrition are also fundamental components of self-care, ensuring your body has the resources it needs to function optimally.

As the chapter closes, reflect on how resilience intertwines with every aspect of life. Embracing its principles can transform how you approach challenges, fostering a sense of empowerment and vitality. Resilience is not just a trait but a lifestyle, one that supports longevity and enhances your quality of life. With these tools, you're poised to navigate the complexities of life with confidence, paving the way for healthier, happier years ahead.

6

HABIT 6: 10 PRIMARY BIOLOGICAL AGE FACTORS THAT ARE UNDERSTOOD TO BE REVERSIBLE

Imagine if the ticking of your biological clock could be recalibrated, so you feel as vibrant and youthful in your later years as you did in your prime. This isn't just an enticing fantasy; it's a possibility grounded in the latest scientific research. We're diving into the realm of biological age factors that can be not only slowed but reversed. These factors hold the key to unlocking a future where aging isn't an inevitable decline, but a state we can manage and even improve.

PINEAL CLOCK

The pineal gland, nestled deep within your brain, serves as your body's master clock, orchestrating the symphony of your circadian rhythms and the dance of hormones and neurotransmitters that guide your daily cycle. This tiny, yet powerful gland produces melatonin, a hormone pivotal in regulating sleep and wakefulness, among other functions. Melatonin production peaks during the dark hours and dwindles as daylight emerges, a process intricately linked to the suprachiasmatic nucleus (SCN), which acts as the brain's central timekeeper. As we age, however, melatonin levels decline significantly, leading to disruptions in sleep patterns and other circadian-dependent processes. This decline isn't merely an inconvenience; it signals to various systems in the body that aging is underway.

The breakdown of the pineal clock can have far-reaching effects, setting off a cascade of aging signals throughout the body. This disruption has been linked to increased risks of metabolic disorders, immune dysfunction, and even neurodegenerative diseases. The importance of maintaining a robust circadian rhythm cannot be overstated, as it influences everything from your mood to your cellular repair processes. Restoring the function of this clock through melatonin supplementation has shown promise in rejuvenating the pineal gland. By supporting melatonin levels, you can help realign your body's internal clock, potentially reversing some age-related changes and improving overall health and wellness.

Incorporating practices that promote healthy pineal function is essential for age reversal. Regular exposure to natural light during the day, especially in the morning, can help set your circadian rhythm, while minimizing light exposure at night can prevent melatonin suppression. Alongside these lifestyle adjustments, melatonin supplementation might serve as a potent tool in your anti-aging arsenal. Its antioxidant properties extend beyond circadian regulation, offering protective benefits against oxidative stress, a major contributor to aging. By embracing these strategies, you can support your pineal clock in maintaining a youthful biological age and enhancing your quality of life.

Reflection Section: Assessing Your Circadian Habits

Consider your daily routines and how they might be impacting your pineal function. Reflect on the following:

- **Morning Light Exposure:** Do you spend time outside in natural light shortly after waking? If not, how can you incorporate this into your routine?
- **Evening Light Habits:** Are you exposed to bright lights or screens close to bedtime? What changes can you make to reduce this exposure?
- **Sleep Environment:** Is your sleep environment conducive to good rest, with minimal light and noise? What improvements can you implement?

By reflecting on these questions, you can identify areas for improvement, optimizing your circadian habits to support a healthier, more youthful biological age.

THYMIC INVOLUTION

The thymus gland, nestled beneath your breastbone, plays a pivotal role in your immune system's ability to fend off infections and diseases. This gland is responsible for the maturation of T-cells, which are crucial defenders against pathogens. However, beginning around the age of thirty, the thymus starts to undergo a process known as involution. What this means is that the gland gradually shrinks and becomes less effective, its once-active tissue slowly replaced by adipose (fat) tissue. By the time many individuals reach sixty-five, the thymus has significantly diminished in function, leading to a decreased output of naïve T-cells. This decline contributes to the aging immune system's vulnerability, presenting a heightened risk of infections and illnesses that the body once easily combated.

The process of thymic involution is not merely a passive consequence of aging but a significant factor in the body's declining ability to mount effective immune responses. The loss of thymic tissue means that fewer new T-cells are produced, which gradually weakens the immune system's capacity to recognize and eliminate new threats. This decline in immune function is associated with increased morbidity and mortality in older adults. However, research into the mechanisms of thymic involution suggests that this process may not be entirely irreversible. Therapeutic interventions, such as the use of cytokines like interleukin 7 (IL-7) and keratinocyte growth factor (KGF), have shown promise in rejuvenating thymic function. These cytokines stimulate thymopoiesis, the production of T-cells, offering a potential pathway to bolster immune competence and extend health span.

Moreover, recent studies have explored the potential of sex steroid ablation (SSA) therapies to reverse thymic atrophy. By temporarily reducing the influence of sex hormones, researchers have observed a resurgence in thymic activity, leading to enhanced immune recovery. While these interventions are still largely in the experimental stages, they offer a glimpse into the possibilities of reversing thymic involution. Another avenue being explored is lifestyle modifications, which include a balanced diet rich in antioxidants, regular physical activity, and stress reduction techniques. These can support immune health by reducing oxidative stress and inflammation, both of which contribute to thymic decline. Engaging in regular exercise, in particular, has been shown to enhance immune function by promoting circulation and increasing the production of immune cells throughout the body.

Addressing thymic involution involves a multifaceted approach that includes emerging therapies and lifestyle choices. As research continues, the potential to restore thymic function and improve immune resilience grows more promising. By understanding and targeting this process, you can take proactive steps to support your immune health, potentially reversing one of the key drivers of biological aging.

BLOOD SIGNALING AND TRANSCRIPTION

Imagine the bloodstream as a vast communication network, constantly transmitting signals that orchestrate the complex symphony of cellular processes. Among these signals are age-related molecules that convey messages to the body's 100 trillion cells, nudging them toward aging. This understanding comes from pioneering experiments with heterochronic parabiosis, where the circulatory systems of young and old animals are connected. The results were astounding. Young blood appeared to rejuvenate older animals, while the older blood accelerated aging in young ones. This suggests that youthfulness and aging are influenced by systemic factors circulating in the blood, which can potentially be modulated or even reversed.

The implications of these findings are profound. They hint at the existence of specific factors in young blood that can activate genes associated with rejuvenation and repair. Conversely, the presence of certain signaling molecules in older blood may promote aging by altering transcriptional activities at the cellular level. These molecules influence gene expression, which in turn affects cellular functions such as metabolism, growth, and repair. By altering these signals, we might unlock new pathways to age reversal. The rejuvenating effects observed in animal studies have spurred interest in identifying these factors, with the goal of developing therapies that can mimic the beneficial effects of young blood.

Researchers are delving into the molecular underpinnings of these phenomena, aiming to isolate the specific components responsible for these effects. Understanding the mechanisms of blood signaling and transcription may lead to innovative treatments that can delay or reverse age-related decline in humans. Scientists are particularly interested in how these factors might affect stem cell function and tissue regeneration, areas crucial for maintaining youthful vitality. The potential to rejuvenate the immune system, enhance cognitive function, and improve muscle strength underscores the transformative power of manipulating blood signaling pathways.

As we explore these possibilities, it becomes clear that the future of age reversal lies not only in the laboratory but also in our ability to apply these insights to human health. While the exact molecular players remain elusive, the promise of blood signaling modulation as a tool for longevity is undeniable. This line of research represents a frontier with the potential to redefine how we approach aging, transforming it from an inevitable decline to a process we can influence. The path forward involves harnessing these insights to create interventions that promote healthy aging, ultimately extending both lifespan and health span.

INFLAMMAGING

Inflammaging is a concept that encapsulates the chronic, low-grade inflammation often associated with aging. Unlike acute inflammation, which is your body's immediate response to injury or infection, inflammaging persists quietly, causing ongoing damage to tissues and cells. Over time, this insidious inflammation contributes to a range of age-related diseases, including arthritis, cardiovascular disease, and even some forms of cancer. The persistent inflammation results from an overactive immune response that, instead of protecting the body, leads to its gradual deterioration. As we age, our immune system becomes less adept at differentiating between foreign invaders and the body's own cells, which can lead to this chronic inflammatory state.

This constant state of inflammation accelerates the aging process by promoting tissue degeneration. As tissues break down, they release pro-inflammatory substances that further fuel the cycle of inflammation, creating a vicious loop that is difficult to interrupt. The immune cells involved in this process, such as macrophages and T-cells, become dysregulated, losing their ability to appropriately respond to threats. This dysregulation, combined with an increase in inflammatory cytokines, damages tissues and impairs the function of various organs, contributing to the overall decline in health seen with aging.

Recent research suggests that lifestyle changes can mitigate the effects of inflammaging. Diet plays a crucial role, with anti-inflammatory foods such as fruits, vegetables, nuts, and fish providing nutrients that can counteract inflammation. These foods are rich in antioxidants and omega-3 fatty acids, which help reduce the production of inflammatory cytokines. Regular physical activity also helps by improving circulation and promoting the release of anti-inflammatory substances. Additionally, stress management techniques like mindfulness and meditation can lower stress hormones that exacerbate inflammation.

Understanding inflammaging provides a pathway to interventions that can slow down, or even reverse, the damage caused by chronic inflammation. By addressing the root causes and symptoms, you can potentially improve your quality of life as you age. This involves adopting healthier lifestyle habits and staying informed about emerging therapies that target inflammation at the cellular level. The exploration of anti-inflammatory drugs and natural supplements continues to offer promising avenues for reducing inflammaging's impact, representing a significant step forward in age reversal research.

EPIGENETIC CLOCK

The concept of the epigenetic clock is a fascinating area of study that highlights how your genes are influenced by more than just the DNA sequence you inherit. Epigenetics involves changes to your DNA, RNA, or proteins that regulate gene expression without altering the underlying genetic code. These modifications are like switches that turn genes on or off, impacting how your body functions and ages. What's intriguing is that these changes aren't set in stone—they are dynamic and can be influenced by factors like diet, stress, and environmental exposure. Essentially, while your genetic code provides the blueprint, epigenetics decides how that blueprint is read and executed.

Your lifestyle choices play a significant role in shaping your epigenetic landscape. The foods you eat, the amount of physical activity you engage in, and even the quality of your social interactions can leave lasting marks on your epigenome. For instance, consuming a diet rich in fruits, vegetables, and whole grains can foster a pattern of epigenetic modifications that promote health and longevity. Conversely, a diet high in processed foods and sugar might lead to adverse modifications, increasing the risk of chronic diseases. It's a reminder that while you can't change your genetics, you have a degree of control over how those genes are expressed.

The environment you live in also exerts a powerful influence on your epigenetic clock. Pollution, exposure to toxins, and even socioeconomic factors can contribute to harmful modifications that accelerate aging. However, positive interventions like reducing stress through mindfulness or meditation can counteract some of these effects. Furthermore, research suggests that certain compounds in foods, such as polyphenols found in green tea and resveratrol in red wine, can have protective effects on the epigenome, potentially slowing the aging process. This opens up exciting possibilities for dietary and lifestyle interventions that might delay biological aging and improve health outcomes.

Understanding the epigenetic clock underscores the interconnectedness of genetics and lifestyle. By making informed choices, you can potentially influence the way your genes are expressed, possibly delaying the onset of age-related decline. While the field of epigenetics is still evolving, it offers a promising avenue for developing strategies to promote healthy aging. As you navigate life's choices, consider how each decision might reverberate through your epigenome, shaping your biological age and overall wellbeing.

TELOMERE LENGTH

At the very core of our cellular structure, telomeres serve as protective caps at the ends of our chromosomes. Imagine them as the plastic tips at the ends of your shoelaces, preventing them from fraying. Much like those tips, telomeres protect the vital genetic information stored in our DNA. When we are born, these telomeres are at their longest, providing robust protection. However, with each cell division—a routine process for growth, repair, and maintenance—our telomeres lose a tiny portion of their length. This gradual shortening is a natural part of aging, acting as a biological clock that counts down the remaining life span of a cell. Over time, and exacerbated by exposures like oxidative stress and inflammation, telomeres become so short that they can no longer protect chromosomes effectively. This triggers a state known as senescence, where cells lose the ability to divide and function normally, contributing to the onset of age-related decline.

The shortening of telomeres is not just a marker of aging; it is actively involved in the aging process itself. When telomeres become critically short, they can no longer prevent the DNA from being perceived as damaged, leading to cellular dysfunction and the potential activation of damage responses. This can result in the accumulation of senescent cells, which secrete pro-inflammatory factors and other substances that can disrupt tissue function and promote aging. The presence of these cells is associated with the decline of tissue function seen in older age and is linked to various diseases, including cardiovascular disease, diabetes, and certain cancers. Studies have shown that individuals with longer telomeres tend to live longer, healthier lives, underscoring the importance of telomere length in maintaining vitality.

Fortunately, research into the mechanisms of telomere maintenance offers hope for mitigating this process. Strategies to preserve telomere length include lifestyle modifications such as a diet rich in antioxidants, regular physical activity, and stress reduction techniques like meditation. These practices can help reduce oxidative stress and inflammation, which are known to accelerate telomere attrition. Moreover, certain natural compounds, such as polyphenols found in foods like green tea and blueberries, have been shown to have protective effects on telomeres. The enzyme telomerase, which can add length back to telomeres, is also a focus of scientific investigation. While not fully understood, activating telomerase may offer a way to restore telomere length and, by extension, cellular function. Understanding and addressing telomere length offers a promising avenue for extending healthspan and potentially reversing some effects of aging. The intersection of lifestyle, diet, and emerging therapies provides a multifaceted approach to maintaining these crucial chromosome protectors, with the potential to enhance longevity and quality of life.

SENOLYTICS

Consider a bustling city where certain buildings have become decrepit, threatening the structural integrity of their surroundings. This analogy mirrors what happens in our bodies with cellular senescence. As we age, some cells enter a state of senescence, where they stop dividing but don't die off. Instead, they linger, releasing inflammatory signals known as the senescence-associated secretory phenotype (SASP). These signals disrupt the normal function of neighboring cells and tissues, much like how a dilapidated building can affect an entire neighborhood. This process contributes significantly to age-related tissue dysfunction and various chronic conditions, from osteoarthritis to cardiovascular diseases.

Senescent cells, though few in number, have an outsized impact due to their ability to influence systemic aging processes. They create a pro-inflammatory environment that hampers tissue regeneration and accelerates the deterioration of healthy cells, leading to a decline in overall organ function. Their secretions can drive chronic inflammation, a key player in many degenerative diseases. Recent research suggests that by targeting these cells for elimination, we can potentially alleviate these age-related disorders. Enter senolytics—a class of drugs designed to selectively clear senescent cells, thus reducing their harmful burden on the body. This therapeutic approach has shown promising results in preclinical studies, where removing senescent cells in animal models improved physical function, extended lifespan, and even rejuvenated tissues.

The potential of senolytics lies in their ability to restore tissue homeostasis by removing the cellular "debris" that clogs the body's repair mechanisms. By clearing these cells, senolytics can enhance the regenerative capacity of tissues, improve metabolic function, and reduce inflammation, leading to a more youthful physiological state. The development of senolytic therapies is still in its infancy, yet it represents a groundbreaking shift in how we might tackle aging. Unlike traditional treatments that focus on symptoms, senolytics aim to address one of the root causes of aging, offering hope for a future where age-related decline is not a foregone conclusion. This innovative approach has sparked a wave of research focused on identifying effective senolytic compounds and understanding their mechanisms of action, paving the way for potential clinical applications in humans.

EXTRA CELLULAR MATRIX STIFFENING

Think of the extracellular matrix (ECM) as the scaffolding that supports and organizes cells, providing structural integrity to tissues. Composed primarily of collagen and elastin, this matrix ensures that tissues remain flexible and resilient. In youth, the abundance of elastin allows tissues to stretch and recoil, maintaining their shape and function. However, as we age, the production of elastin decreases, while collagen becomes more prevalent. This shift in balance results in the stiffening of the ECM, which can have profound effects on the body. Over time, the reduced elasticity contributes to the rigidity of tissues, which is a hallmark of several age-related diseases. This stiffening is particularly impactful in the cardiovascular system, where it can lead to conditions such as hypertension and atherosclerosis. As the ECM becomes less pliable, blood vessels lose their ability to expand and contract efficiently, putting increased pressure on the heart to maintain circulation.

This process of ECM stiffening is not confined to the cardiovascular system. It affects various organs and tissues, influencing their ability to function optimally. In the lungs, for instance, the decrease in elastin impacts the ability to breathe deeply and efficiently, potentially leading to respiratory issues. Similarly, in the skin, the loss of elastin results in diminished elasticity and the formation of wrinkles, visible signs of aging. The stiffening of the ECM also plays a role in the aging of connective tissues, affecting mobility and leading to joint stiffness. These changes contribute to physical decline and impact the quality of life, as they can limit activity and increase the risk of injury.

While the damage to the ECM is largely considered irreversible, emerging research suggests that certain interventions might help mitigate its effects. Lifestyle choices, such as maintaining a balanced diet rich in antioxidants, can help reduce oxidative stress, a factor that accelerates ECM stiffening. Regular physical activity also supports circulation and promotes the production of factors that maintain tissue health. Additionally, there is growing interest in the potential of therapies aimed at restoring ECM components or inhibiting the enzymes that degrade elastin and collagen. Although these treatments are still in their infancy, they offer hope for slowing the progression of ECM stiffening and its associated health issues. Moreover, understanding the mechanisms behind ECM changes can inform strategies to preserve tissue flexibility, potentially extending the functional lifespan of various organs and systems.

STEM CELL EXHAUSTION

Imagine a bustling city, vibrant and full of life, where buildings are constantly being repaired and upgraded. This city thrives because of its ability to renew itself continuously. In your body, that role is played by stem cells. These remarkable cells have the unique ability to differentiate into specialized cells and replenish other cells, maintaining the dynamic balance of health and repair. Yet, as you age, this regenerative power diminishes—a phenomenon known as stem cell exhaustion. It's as if the city's repair crews are dwindling, leaving buildings to deteriorate over time. Stem cell exhaustion occurs due to accumulated DNA damage, prolonged cellular stress, and the eventual senescence of these pivotal cells. As their numbers and functionality decline, the body's capacity to regenerate tissues and respond to damage diminishes, leading to age-related disorders such as frailty, impaired healing, and increased susceptibility to diseases.

This depletion doesn't just mean fewer stem cells; it also impacts the regenerative capacity of tissues throughout your body. The bone marrow, for instance, is a primary residence for hematopoietic stem cells, which are crucial for producing blood cells. As these stem cells exhaust, the immune system weakens, reducing your body's ability to fend off infections and recover from injuries. Similarly, muscle stem cells, known as satellite cells, lose their potency, resulting in muscle atrophy and decreased strength. This gradual decline is a major contributor to the functional impairments often seen in aging individuals. But what if you could slow or even reverse this exhaustion? Emerging research points to the potential of interventions that could rejuvenate stem cells, thereby restoring their vitality and extending their functional lifespan.

Recent studies suggest that certain lifestyle interventions can have a profound impact on stem cell health. Regular exercise has been shown to stimulate stem cell activity, enhancing their ability to regenerate and repair damaged tissues. A diet rich in antioxidants can also protect stem cells from oxidative damage, which is a significant factor in their decline. Caloric restriction and fasting have been linked to increased stem cell function, potentially delaying the onset of exhaustion. These practices may enhance autophagy, a cellular process that clears damaged components, allowing stem cells to function more efficiently. Additionally, the field of regenerative medicine is exploring novel therapies, such as stem cell transplantation and genetic interventions, aimed at rejuvenating these vital cells. As we continue to understand the intricate mechanisms of stem cell exhaustion, these insights offer a promising pathway to mitigating age-related decline and promoting a healthier, more vibrant life.

CELLULAR METABOLIC EFFICIENCY

Imagine your cells as tiny power plants, each one working tirelessly to convert nutrients into energy. This energy, stored as adenosine triphosphate (ATP), fuels every action your body takes, from a simple breath to the complex firing of neurons in your brain. When your body operates at peak cellular metabolic efficiency (CME), these power plants run smoothly, maximizing energy production while minimizing waste. Achieving CME is akin to fine-tuning an engine to operate with minimal friction and maximal output. The secret to this efficiency lies in the delicate balance of reducing oxidative stress and ensuring high bioavailability of antioxidants.

Oxidative stress occurs when there is an imbalance between free radicals and antioxidants in your body, leading to the potential for cellular damage. This imbalance is like letting rust eat away at your car's engine. However, when antioxidants are abundant and bioavailable, they neutralize free radicals, preventing them from wreaking havoc on your cells. This process preserves cellular integrity and enhances the efficiency of mitochondrial function. Mitochondria, the energy-producing organelles within cells, are particularly sensitive to oxidative stress. By safeguarding them with antioxidants, you ensure they continue to churn out ATP efficiently, supporting overall cell health and vitality.

Antioxidants come in many forms, from vitamins like C and E to compounds like glutathione and coenzyme Q10. These molecules act as scavengers, seeking out and neutralizing free radicals before they can cause damage. But their effectiveness depends not just on quantity but also on bioavailability—the ease with which they are absorbed and utilized by the body. This is why dietary choices are crucial. Consuming a diet rich in colorful fruits and vegetables, nuts, and seeds provides a spectrum of antioxidants that are readily absorbed. Incorporating foods like berries, spinach, and nuts can boost your cells' defenses, ensuring that your body's metabolic processes run smoothly and efficiently, slowing the aging process.

As inflammation is a natural byproduct of oxidative stress, reducing it further enhances CME. With less inflammation, your cells can focus on performing their functions rather than repairing themselves from damage. This not only supports longevity but also enhances your quality of life, allowing you to maintain energy levels and reduce the risk of age-related diseases. In essence, optimizing cellular metabolic efficiency is about creating an environment where your cells can thrive, providing you with the vitality and resilience needed for a healthy, vibrant life.

10 PRIMARY BIOLOGICAL AGE FACTOR FORMULATIONS AND RECOMMENDED DOSAGE

Implementing the habits discussed requires not only understanding, but also precise application. For many of the supplements and interventions, a consistent routine is key. Take, for instance, the regimented use of specific solutions designed to support your body's biological age reversal. The recommended formulations are available from Extended Longevity Inc. https://www.extended longevity.com/store

These 10 Primary Biological Age Factors involve taking one milliliter (1 ml) orally of each daily. Administering nine droppers in the morning before meals capitalizes on your body's heightened receptivity to nutrients and activators when it is in a fasting state. This timing takes advantage of the natural metabolic processes that are more active in the morning, setting a positive tone for your body's functions throughout the day.

In the evening, the use of Pinetonal is suggested. This is taken as one dropper full before bedtime. The rationale behind this timing is to align with your body's circadian rhythms, facilitating processes like cellular repair, detoxification, and the regulation of sleep hormones. Taking supplements at night can complement your body's natural restorative activities. The option to take these supplements under the tongue or with water provides flexibility, accommodating personal preferences and ensuring ease of integration into your daily routine. This sublingual method can enhance absorption, ensuring that the active compounds enter the bloodstream more directly and efficiently.

IMPORTANT: The laboratory basis of these formulations is alcohol. When they arrive, open the lid of each container and allow to sit in the open air for several hours. This allows the alcohol to evaporate. Another method is to place each container in warm water (without boiling) which speeds up the alcohol evaporation.

This structured approach to supplementation is more than just a routine; it is a calculated method to support your body's intricate systems as they work to reverse aging. Consistency in dosage not only ensures that your body receives a steady supply of vital nutrients and compounds but also helps to maintain optimal levels of these substances. Over time, this practice may contribute to improved cellular function, better energy levels, and enhanced vitality. It is a simple yet powerful tool in the quest to age not just gracefully, but strategically. As you incorporate these practices, remember that the journey of age reversal is as much about the habits you cultivate as it is about the tools you employ.

In the next chapter, we will explore how to integrate these habits seamlessly into your daily life, ensuring that the knowledge you've gained translates into lasting transformation and enhanced well-being.

7

BONUS HABIT: INTEGRATING AGE-REVERSING HABITS INTO DAILY LIFE

Have you ever found yourself struggling to incorporate new habits into your daily routine despite knowing their benefits? The secret to seamlessly integrating these habits lies in a method called habit stacking. It's a technique that uses the power of existing routines to build new, positive behaviors without overwhelming your schedule. Imagine the ease of pairing a new habit with something you already do effortlessly, like sipping your morning coffee or winding down at night. Habit stacking leverages the brain's tendency to follow established patterns, making it easier to introduce changes that can reverse your biological age.

Habit stacking is a strategic approach to behavior change, where new habits are linked to established ones, creating a chain of actions that flow naturally. This concept taps into the trigger-behavior-reward cycle, a fundamental principle in habit formation. The trigger is the cue that initiates the behavior, while the behavior itself is the action you want to adopt. The reward reinforces the behavior, encouraging you to repeat it. By attaching a new habit to an existing one, you utilize the established trigger as a cue for the new behavior, making it easier to remember and execute. This process takes advantage of the brain's neural connections that are already in place, strengthening them with each repetition. The role of cues in habit initiation is crucial; they act as reminders that prompt you to act without conscious effort, turning desirable behaviors into automatic responses over time.

For instance, consider the simple act of making coffee in the morning. By associating this routine with a brief meditation session, you create a habit stack that integrates mindfulness into your daily life without requiring additional time. As you wait for your coffee to brew, take a moment to sit quietly and focus on your breath, setting a calm tone for the day ahead. Similarly, try pairing a short mindfulness exercise with your daily walk. As you step outside, consciously engage your senses—notice the sights, sounds, and scents around you. This practice enhances your walk and anchors you in the present moment, reducing stress and promoting mental clarity. These examples illustrate how habit stacking can transform mundane routines into powerful tools for age reversal.

To effectively implement habit stacking, begin by mapping out your daily routines to identify opportunities for new habits. Look for moments in your day that occur consistently, such as brushing your teeth or preparing meals. These are ideal anchors for habit stacking because they provide reliable cues. Once you've identified potential triggers, brainstorm new habits you wish to incorporate, ensuring they are specific and actionable. For example, you might decide to perform a series of stretching exercises while brushing your teeth, using the sink as a support for balance. This integrates physical activity into your routine without disrupting your schedule. Similarly, consider adding gratitude journaling to your bedtime ritual. Before turning off the lights, take a few minutes to reflect on the day's positive moments, fostering a sense of gratitude and contentment. By linking these actions to existing habits, you create a seamless flow that supports long-term consistency.

Interactive Element: Habit Stacking Worksheet

Use the worksheet below to identify your current habits and plan new habit stacks:

1. List three daily activities you perform consistently (e.g., morning coffee, lunchtime break, evening relaxation).
2. Identify three new habits you'd like to incorporate (e.g., meditation, journaling, stretching).
3. Match each new habit with an existing activity to form a habit stack.
4. Write down your new habit stacks and keep them visible as a reminder.

Developing personalized routines through habit stacking requires thoughtful consideration of your lifestyle and preferences. Start small, focusing on one or two habit stacks at a time to avoid feeling overwhelmed. As these new habits become ingrained, gradually introduce additional stacks to further enhance your routine. Remember, the key to success lies in consistency and patience. By leveraging the power of existing habits, you create a strong foundation for sustainable change. This approach supports your journey towards age reversal and fosters a lifestyle that prioritizes health and well-being.

TIME MANAGEMENT STRATEGIES FOR HEALTH PRIORITIZATION

In the whirlwind of modern life, effectively managing your time is not just about getting things done; it's about carving out space for the activities that matter most to your health and well-being. Prioritizing health goals amidst a busy schedule requires intentional time management. This means balancing the demands of work with personal obligations, all while making room for exercise, meal preparation, and relaxation. Time management isn't just a skill; it's a necessity for those who aim to incorporate age-reversing habits into their daily routines. By allocating time to these practices, you ensure that your health remains at the forefront, not an afterthought.

A powerful technique for embedding health activities into your schedule is time blocking. This method involves dividing your day into specific blocks of time, each dedicated to a particular task or activity. By assigning fixed times for exercise sessions, you create a non-negotiable appointment with yourself, much like a business meeting you wouldn't cancel. Similarly, planning meal preparation times ensures that you have healthy options readily available, reducing the temptation for quick but unhealthy alternatives. Time blocking enhances adherence to your health goals by providing structure and reducing the mental clutter of deciding what to do next. It transforms good intentions into actionable steps, making it easier to stick to your commitments.

To efficiently organize your time, leverage the power of digital calendars with reminders. These tools help you visualize your day, ensuring that nothing falls through the cracks. Setting alerts for health breaks during work can prompt you to step away from your desk, stretch, and recharge, preventing burnout and maintaining productivity. The Pomodoro technique, a time management method that involves working in focused intervals followed by short breaks, can be particularly effective. This approach enhances concentration and ensures that you regularly take time to relax, which is crucial for sustaining energy throughout the day. These tools and techniques make it easier to balance the demands of life while keeping your health a priority.

Procrastination is a common obstacle in maintaining health routines, but several strategies can help you overcome it. Breaking tasks into smaller, manageable steps can make daunting activities feel more achievable. For instance, if the thought of a long workout is overwhelming, start with a short 10-minute session. This small step often leads to more, as momentum builds with action. Rewarding yourself for progress can also boost motivation. Celebrating milestones, no matter how small, reinforces positive behavior and keeps you moving forward. This could be as simple as enjoying a favorite activity after completing a workout, or treating yourself to a new book after a week of meal prepping. By focusing on progress rather than perfection, you create a positive feedback loop that encourages continued effort.

Interactive Element: Time Management Audit

Take a moment to evaluate how you currently spend your time. Identify areas where you can allocate more time to health practices. Write down your daily activities, highlighting those that align with your health goals. Look for patterns or habits that could be adjusted to make room for new practices. Consider substituting a less productive activity, like excessive screen time, with a health-focused one. This audit helps you understand your current time usage and identify opportunities for improvement.

Incorporating these strategies into your life requires commitment and consistency, but the rewards are well worth the effort. By effectively managing your time, you create a lifestyle that supports your age-reversing goals, ensuring that health becomes a sustained priority rather than a fleeting intention.

MEAL PLANNING AND PREPARATION FOR NUTRITIONAL SUCCESS

In the vast landscape of health and wellness, meal planning emerges as a cornerstone for achieving nutritional goals and reducing daily stress. When you take the time to plan your meals in advance, you do more than just ensure balanced nutrient intake; you cultivate a sense of control over your diet, minimizing the impulsive choices that often derail your efforts. Picture this: instead of scrambling to assemble a meal at the last minute, you have a pre-planned menu tailored to your nutritional needs. This foresight not only supports your aim to maintain a balanced diet but also alleviates the stress of daily decision-making. By thoughtfully planning your meals, you provide yourself with a clear path to follow, eliminating the uncertainty that often leads to unhealthy eating habits.

To embark on a successful meal planning journey, start with a structured approach. Begin by creating weekly menus that reflect your dietary goals and preferences. Consider incorporating a variety of food groups to ensure a comprehensive nutrient profile. Once your menu is set, engage in batch cooking. This involves preparing larger quantities of food that can be portioned and stored for future meals. By cooking in bulk, you save time during the week and reduce the temptation to opt for less healthy options when time is tight. Portioning meals into individual containers allows for easy access and control over portion sizes, which is vital for maintaining a balanced diet. This method ensures that every meal you consume aligns with your nutritional intentions, supporting both your health and age-reversal goals.

Efficiency in the kitchen is crucial, especially for those with demanding schedules. To streamline meal preparation, consider time-saving techniques such as cooking in bulk for freezer storage. By preparing and freezing meals ahead of time, you create a reservoir of healthy options that can be quickly reheated and enjoyed. This saves time on busy days and ensures that you always have nutritious meals at your fingertips. Pre-chopping ingredients is another practical tip that can significantly reduce prep time. By washing, chopping, and storing vegetables and other ingredients in advance, you can quickly assemble meals without the hassle of starting from scratch each time you cook. These techniques minimize the effort required to maintain a healthy diet, making meal preparation a more manageable part of your routine.

In today's digital age, numerous tools and resources are available to facilitate meal planning. Apps like Mealime provide personalized recipe suggestions and generate grocery lists based on your preferences, simplifying the planning process. These apps offer the convenience of having meal ideas and shopping lists at your fingertips, reducing the mental load of planning your diet. Grocery list generators further enhance efficiency by ensuring you have all the necessary ingredients for your planned meals, minimizing the need for last-minute trips to the store. By leveraging these resources, you can streamline your meal planning process, making it easier to stick to your nutritional goals and support your age-reversing habits.

CREATING A PERSONAL WELLNESS SPACE AT HOME

Creating a dedicated wellness space at home is more than just a trend; it's a commitment to your health and well-being. This space serves as a sanctuary where you can focus on exercise, meditation, or simply taking a moment to breathe. By having a designated area for your health practices, you enhance consistency and make it easier to stick to your routines. Visual cues, such as yoga mats or meditation cushions, reinforce these habits, reminding you of your commitment every time you see them. The importance of having a personal wellness space cannot be overstated; it acts as a physical reminder of your health priorities, encouraging regular engagement with your age-reversing habits.

Setting up an effective wellness environment requires thoughtful planning. Start by selecting a quiet, clutter-free area in your home. This space should be free from distractions, allowing you to focus entirely on your health practices. Consider incorporating calming elements like plants or candles, which can enhance the ambiance and promote relaxation. Plants purify the air and create a serene atmosphere, while candles can provide gentle lighting that soothes the senses. These elements transform an ordinary corner of your home into a retreat where you can recharge and rejuvenate. Whether it's a spare room or just a small nook, the key is to create a space that feels inviting and dedicated to your well-being.

For those with limited space, creating a multipurpose wellness environment is both practical and achievable. Transforming a corner for yoga and meditation can be as simple as laying down a mat and adding a few cushions. Versatile furniture, such as a foldable table or a bookshelf that doubles as a makeshift altar, can serve multiple purposes, maximizing the functionality of your space. This adaptability ensures that your wellness area can accommodate various activities, from exercise to mindfulness, without requiring extensive renovations or investments. By thinking creatively about your space, you can ensure it meets your needs without compromising on comfort or utility.

Personalization and comfort are crucial when designing your wellness space. Choose soothing colors and decorations that resonate with you, creating an environment that's not only functional but also visually appealing. Soft blues or greens can evoke a sense of calm, while warm tones might provide a more invigorating atmosphere. Incorporate personal items that inspire you, such as artwork, photographs, or meaningful objects. These touches make the space uniquely yours, fostering a deeper connection to your health practices. Comfort is key, so ensure your space has elements that allow you to fully relax and engage with your routines, whether through comfortable seating or plush textiles.

A well-curated wellness space acts as a catalyst for personal growth and self-care. By deliberately carving out a part of your home for health-focused activities, you prioritize your well-being in a tangible way. This intentionality not only supports your physical health but also nurtures mental and emotional resilience. Engaging with your wellness space regularly can lead to a more balanced lifestyle, where health practices become seamlessly integrated into your daily life. Each time you step into this space, you're reminded of your commitment to self-care, reinforcing the habits that support your age-reversal journey. This space becomes a personal haven, offering solace and inspiration amidst the demands of everyday life.

ACCOUNTABILITY PARTNERS: STAYING ON TRACK TOGETHER

Have you ever noticed how much easier it is to stick to a commitment when someone else is counting on you? This is the power of having an accountability partner. An accountability partner is someone who shares your health goals and supports you in achieving them. The concept is simple yet profoundly effective: two people working together, providing mutual support and encouragement, to stay committed to their health activities. When you have someone by your side, tracking progress becomes a shared journey, and the obstacles that seemed insurmountable alone become manageable. The presence of a partner can transform your approach to health, making it not just a personal endeavor but a collaborative one.

The benefits of accountability relationships are vast and impactful. First and foremost, having a support system increases your commitment to health activities. When you know someone else is involved in your goals, you're more likely to stick to your plans, whether it's attending a fitness class or following a nutrition plan. This shared responsibility fosters a sense of obligation not just to yourself but to your partner as well. Moreover, during challenging times, when motivation wanes or setbacks occur, an accountability partner serves as a source of encouragement. They can offer perspective, celebrate your successes, and remind you of your progress when you're feeling discouraged. This emotional support is invaluable, helping you stay focused and resilient in the face of adversity.

Selecting the right accountability partner is crucial for mutual success. It's important to choose someone whose health goals and interests align with your own. This alignment ensures that both of you are working towards similar objectives, making it easier to share strategies and celebrate milestones together. Additionally, establishing clear communication channels is essential. Regular check-ins, whether in person or through virtual platforms, help maintain the momentum and keep both partners informed about each other's progress. Open and honest communication allows you to address challenges, share insights, and adjust goals as needed. This collaborative approach strengthens the partnership and enhances the likelihood of achieving your health goals.

To actively engage with your accountability partner, consider incorporating activities that foster collaboration and motivation. Regular check-ins and progress updates are fundamental in keeping the partnership dynamic. These can be scheduled weekly or bi-weekly, providing opportunities to discuss achievements, setbacks, and adjustments to your plans. Joint participation in health activities can also be highly beneficial. Whether it's attending a yoga class, going for a walk, or preparing healthy meals together, these shared experiences reinforce your commitment and make health activities more enjoyable. By turning individual pursuits into shared endeavors, you create a supportive environment that encourages both partners to stay on track.

Incorporating accountability into your health routine can be transformative. It shifts the focus from solitary effort to collective progress, providing the structure and motivation needed to overcome obstacles and achieve lasting change. The partnership fosters a sense of camaraderie and shared responsibility, making health goals more attainable and sustainable. By choosing the right partner and actively engaging in the process, you can enhance your journey towards age reversal, ensuring that your efforts are supported and celebrated along the way. This collaborative approach not only enriches your personal health experience but also strengthens the bonds of friendship and shared purpose, creating a foundation for lifelong wellness.

TECHNOLOGY TOOLS: LEVERAGING APPS FOR HEALTH MONITORING

In today's digital age, technology has become a powerful ally in managing health and supporting age-reversing habits. The ability to track progress, set goals, and receive reminders all through your smartphone or wearable device can transform the way you approach your health journey. Digital tools provide you with the ability to monitor various health metrics, ensuring you're on track to meet your goals. Whether it's tracking your daily steps or monitoring your heart rate, these tools offer insights that were once only available in a clinical setting. They help you visualize your progress, celebrate milestones, and adjust your strategies as needed. With these digital assistants, staying on top of your health becomes less of a chore and more of an integrated part of your lifestyle.

Many health apps offer specialized functions that cater to different aspects of health management. Fitness tracking apps, like MyFitnessPal, allow you to log your workouts and track your caloric intake, giving you a comprehensive view of your physical activity and nutrition. These apps often include features like calorie counters and exercise logs, making it easy to stay accountable. Sleep monitoring apps, such as Sleep Cycle, analyze your sleep patterns and provide feedback on how to improve your rest. By understanding how well you sleep, you can make informed decisions about your nighttime routine, ensuring you get the restorative rest necessary for optimal health. These apps are designed to fit seamlessly into your routine, providing valuable data without overwhelming your day.

Wearable technology further enhances your ability to monitor health metrics in real time. Devices like fitness trackers and smartwatches have become ubiquitous, offering features that track everything from steps taken to heart rate variability. These wearables provide immediate feedback, allowing you to adjust your activity levels on the fly. Biofeedback devices take this a step further by offering insights into physiological processes such as breathing patterns and stress levels. By providing real-time data, these devices empower you to make immediate adjustments to your lifestyle, enhancing your ability to maintain balance and well-being. The integration of wearable technology into daily life makes health monitoring more accessible and less intrusive, allowing you to focus on living rather than tracking.

Selecting the right apps and devices requires consideration of several factors to ensure they meet your needs effectively. User-friendliness is paramount; the app should be intuitive and easy to navigate, ensuring that you can use it without frustration. Customization options are also important, allowing you to tailor the app to your specific goals and preferences. Data privacy is another critical aspect to consider. As these apps often collect sensitive health information, ensuring that they have robust data protection measures in place is essential. Look for apps with transparent privacy policies and those that allow you to control what information is shared. By selecting the right tools, you can enhance your health journey while safeguarding your personal information.

The role of technology in health management cannot be overstated. It provides a bridge between intention and action, offering the tools needed to track progress and make informed decisions. By leveraging these digital tools, you can enhance your ability to integrate age-reversing habits into your daily routine, ensuring that you stay on track and motivated. As you become more familiar with these technologies, you'll find that they offer not just data but insights that can transform your approach to health. Embracing the possibilities of technology allows you to take control of your well-being, creating a more informed and empowered path towards age reversal.

YOUR CHANCE TO MAKE A DIFFERENCE

Now that you're equipped to begin your own transformative health journey, you're also equipped to help others along on theirs. Please take a moment to help more people find this book so that they, too, can improve their health and reverse their biological age.

Simply by sharing your honest opinion of this book and a little about your own experience, you'll show new readers where they can find it and inspire them to take this journey for themselves.

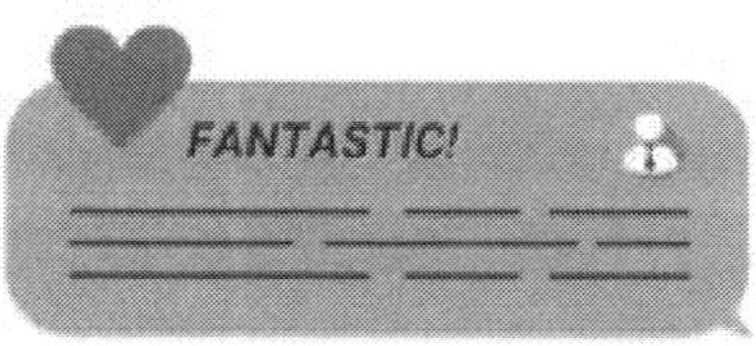

Thank you so much for your support. I wish you a long, healthy, and happy life.

Scan the QR code below.

CONCLUSION

As we come to the end of this transformative journey, I want to emphasize the power you hold to reclaim your vitality and reverse your biological age. Throughout these pages, we've explored the six essential habits that form the foundation of a youthful, vibrant life. From the intricacies of nutrigenomics to the rejuvenating effects of sleep, each habit plays a crucial role in optimizing your health and longevity.

Nutrition and diet lie at the heart of age reversal. By understanding how food interacts with your genes, you can harness the power of nutrigenomics to support cellular health. Antioxidant-rich foods like berries, herbal tea, and dark leafy greens combat oxidative stress, while intermittent fasting triggers cellular repair mechanisms. These dietary strategies work synergistically to promote longevity and vitality.

Movement is another key pillar of youthfulness. Engaging in a diverse range of exercise modalities, from high-intensity interval training to strength training and mind-body practices like yoga and tai chi, enhances cardiovascular health, maintains muscle mass, and promotes mental well-being. By incorporating these activities into your daily life, you tap into your body's innate ability to regenerate and thrive.

The impact of healthy relationships and meaningful activities cannot be overstated. Cultivating strong social connections, engaging with your community, and pursuing purposeful endeavors nourish your soul and contribute to a longer, happier life. Prioritizing these aspects of well-being is just as important as attending to your physical health.

Sleep, often overlooked, is a critical component of age reversal. By optimizing your sleep cycles, creating a sleep-conducive environment, and aligning with your circadian rhythms, you allow your body to repair, rejuvenate, and maintain its youthful resilience. Prioritizing restful sleep is an investment in your vitality and longevity.

Stress management is another essential piece of the longevity puzzle. Chronic stress accelerates aging, but by cultivating mindfulness, practicing breathing techniques, and building resilience, you can mitigate its impact. These strategies not only promote mental well-being but also support cellular health and overall longevity.

The field of nutritional science continues to unveil powerful compounds that can help reverse aging. Omega-3 fatty acids, polyphenols, and vitamin D are just a few examples of nutrients that support cellular health and promote youthfulness. By incorporating these nutrients into your diet, you provide your body with the building blocks it needs to thrive.

Integrating these habits into your daily life may seem daunting, but with strategies like habit stacking, effective time management, and creating supportive environments, you can make this transformative journey a seamless part of your routine. Remember, small steps lead to significant changes over time.

As we look to the future, innovative practices and emerging research offer exciting possibilities for extending lifespan and enhancing vitality. From senolytics that clear aging cells to gene therapies and personalized medicine, the field of age reversal is rapidly evolving. By staying informed and open to these advancements, you position yourself at the forefront of this transformative movement.

The vision that biological age can be effectively reversed is not just a dream—it's a reality supported by rigorous scientific research. The practical strategies and insights provided in this book empower you to take control of your health and reclaim your youthfulness. By implementing these evidence-based habits, you can experience the profound benefits of a revitalized mind and body.

I encourage you to start integrating these habits into your life today. Each small step you take brings you closer to your goal of optimal health and vitality. Embrace the transformative power of these practices and witness the incredible changes that unfold.

As you embark on this journey, remember that you are not alone. Join a community of like-minded individuals who are also committed to reversing their biological age. Share your progress, support one another, and celebrate the victories along the way. Together, we can create a world where vibrant health and longevity are the norm, not the exception.

I leave you with this final thought: your body is a remarkable, resilient vessel capable of incredible transformation. By nurturing it with the right habits and mindset, you unlock its innate potential for healing, regeneration, and vitality. Embrace this truth, and let it guide you on your path to a life filled with boundless energy, joy, and youthfulness.

Thank you for joining me on this transformative journey. I am honored to have been your guide, and I am excited to see the incredible transformations you will achieve. Remember, the power to reverse your biological age lies within you. Seize it, cherish it, and let it shine brightly for all to see.

REFERENCES

"Health Quotes." Inspirational Quotes at BrainyQuote. Accessed March 11, 2025. https://www.brainyquote.com/topics/health-quotes.

Nutrigenomics at the Interface of Aging, Lifespan, and Cancer ... https://pubmed.ncbi.nlm.nih.gov/27558581/

Plant Fortification of the Diet for Anti-Ageing Effects: A Review https://pmc.ncbi.nlm.nih.gov/articles/PMC7601865/

Intermittent fasting and longevity: From animal models to ... https://www.sciencedirect.com/science/article/abs/pii/S1568163724000928

Fermented Foods, Health and the Gut Microbiome - PMC https://pmc.ncbi.nlm.nih.gov/articles/PMC9003261/

Mayo Clinic discovers high-intensity aerobic training can ... https://newsnetwork.mayoclinic.org/discussion/mayo-clinic-discovers-high-intensity-aerobic-training-can-reverse-aging-processes-in-adults/

Strength training: Get stronger, leaner, healthier - Mayo Clinic https://www.mayoclinic.org/healthy-lifestyle/fitness/in-depth/strength-training/art-20046670

Aging: Improving flexibility may help people live longer https://www.medicalnewstoday.com/articles/being-more-flexible-help-people-live-longer

Exercising with arthritis: Improve your joint pain and stiffness https://www.mayoclinic.org/diseases-conditions/arthritis/in-depth/arthritis/art-20047971

Social relationships and physiological determinants of ... https://pmc.ncbi.nlm.nih.gov/articles/PMC4725506/

3 health benefits of volunteering https://www.mayoclinichealthsystem.org/hometown-health/speaking-of-health/3-health-benefits-of-volunteering

Sense of Purpose in Life and Healthier Cognitive Aging https://pmc.ncbi.nlm.nih.gov/articles/PMC8987293/

Volunteering and its Surprising Benefits https://www.helpguide.org/mental-health/wellbeing/volunteering-and-its-surprising-benefits

Sleep stages and memory https://www.health.harvard.edu/healthbeat/sleep-stages-and-memory

Everything You Need to Create the Bedroom of Your Dreams https://www.healthline.com/health/healthy-sleep/ultimate-guide-for-turning-your-bedroom-into-a-sleep-sanctuary

Importance of circadian timing for aging and longevity https://www.nature.com/articles/s41467-021-22922-6

9 Supplements That May Help You Sleep (According to Studies) https://www.goodrx.com/conditions/insomnia/supplements-for-sleep

Stress, Inflammation and Aging - PMC https://pmc.ncbi.nlm.nih.gov/articles/PMC3428505/

Mindfulness meditation: A research-proven way to reduce ... https://www.apa.org/topics/mindfulness/meditation

10 Breathing Exercises to Try When You're Feeling Stressed https://www.healthline.com/health/breathing-exercise

Nurtured by nature https://www.apa.org/monitor/2020/04/nurtured-nature

Physiology of the Pineal Gland and Melatonin - NCBI https://www.ncbi.nlm.nih.gov/books/NBK550972/

Thymic involution and immune reconstitution - PMC https://pmc.ncbi.nlm.nih.gov/articles/PMC2750859/

Aging insights from heterochronic parabiosis models - Nature https://www.nature.com/articles/s41514-024-00166-0

Telomere dysfunction in ageing and age-related diseases https://www.nature.com/articles/s41556-022-00842-x

How to Build New Habits by Taking Advantage of Old Ones https://jamesclear.com/habit-stacking

9 Popular Time Management Techniques and Tools | USAHS https://www.usa.edu/blog/time-management-techniques/

Best Meal-Planning Apps of 2024 (Tested and Reviewed) https://www.cosmopolitan.com/lifestyle/g44052513/best-meal-planning-apps/

The Role of Accountability in Achieving Health Goals https://flourishcounselingmd.com/accountability-for-achieving-health-goals

Made in the USA
Monee, IL
05 November 2026

67858591R00070